Volunteers
Palliative Care

Volunteers in Hospice and Palliative Care

A resource for Voluntary Services Managers

SECOND EDITION

Edited by

Ros Scott and Steven Howlett

Advisory Editor

Derek Doyle

With a Foreword by

Barbara Monroe

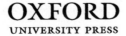

OXFORD
UNIVERSITY PRESS

OXFORD
UNIVERSITY PRESS

Great Clarendon Street, Oxford OX2 6DP

Oxford University Press is a department of the University of Oxford.
It furthers the University's objective of excellence in research, scholarship,
and education by publishing worldwide in

Oxford New York

Auckland Cape Town Dar es Salaam Hong Kong Karachi
Kuala Lumpur Madrid Melbourne Mexico City Nairobi
New Delhi Shanghai Taipei Toronto

With offices in

Argentina Austria Brazil Chile Czech Republic France Greece
Guatemala Hungary Italy Japan Poland Portugal Singapore
South Korea Switzerland Thailand Turkey Ukraine Vietnam

Oxford is a registered trade mark of Oxford University Press
in the UK and in certain other countries

Published in the United States
by Oxford University Press Inc., New York

© Oxford University Press 2009

The moral rights of the author have been asserted
Database right Oxford University Press (maker)

First edition published 2002 (edited by Derek Doyle)
Second edition published 2009

British Library Cataloguing in Publication Data

Data available

Library of Congress Cataloging in Publication Data

Data available

Typeset by Cepha Imaging Private Ltd., Bangalore, India
Printed in Great Britain
on acid-free paper by
the MPG Books Group, Bodmin and King's Lynn

ISBN 978-0-19-954582-7

10 9 8 7 6 5 4 3 2 1

Foreword

Volunteering is firmly embedded in the culture of end-of-life care. In the United Kingdom alone there are over 200 hospices and it is estimated that they benefit from the services of more than 100 000 volunteers, with an economic value at the time of writing of over £110m per annum (Help the Hospices 2006). In Kerala, in Southern India, trained volunteers form the backbone of palliative care service delivery, ensuring a comprehensive community response, supported by professional health carers, despite it being a state with very low per capita income. Volunteering in general is currently the subject of considerable international government interest as attempts are made to stimulate engagement and trust in civic society and to achieve social integration in increasingly multi-ethnic, multi-cultural, multi-faith societies, many with a growing polarization between young and old.

When St Christopher's in London, widely regarded as the first modern hospice, opened in 1967, its Founder Dame Cicely Saunders emphasized that volunteers from the local community would be part of the caring team. She subsequently always mentioned that she enrolled the first volunteers at St Christopher's before the first patient arrived. She believed that institutions alone cannot build communities and understood that volunteers could underpin and respond to the social dimension of many of the issues faced by patients and those close to them. As well as enhancing service provision, volunteers in palliative care services can help by: mobilizing local support, becoming involved in income generation, delivering cost-effective responses to need, ensuring a variety of community representation and normalizing death, dying, and bereavement. When they return to the communities in which they live, volunteers can influence public attitudes and the skills they acquire can contribute to general community well-being and cohesion. Of course, individual volunteers also gain in confidence and skills and reap the benefits of social citizenship. For all these benefits to be realized there must be purposeful and professional volunteer management. Studies increasingly indicate that for volunteer contributions to be effective, high quality recruitment, supervision, support, and training are essential (Field *et al.* 2007, Relf 1998, Rochester 2006). Volunteer services managers must ensure that volunteers have an organizational voice and that their role is owned and valued by all paid staff, the Executive, and the Board. Beyond these immediate building blocks of management, volunteers need to be recognized and rewarded. Their roles must be meaningful and Voluntary Services Managers are likely to become increasingly involved in the development of learning opportunities and accredited qualifications for volunteers. They are also in the vanguard of developing creative responses to changing patterns of volunteering.

Many palliative care services see volunteering opportunities not only as a direct benefit to the organization, but also a way of returning thanks to the community and assisting in developing social capital. There are obvious management challenges to respond to diversity and to ensure that information about volunteering is available to all in a variety of formats and venues, and that it does not rely on word of mouth 'cloning'. It is of interest to note that in the United Kingdom, 37 per cent of refugees and asylum seekers volunteer, often taking their first steps to integrate into U.K. society and prepare the ground for paid employment through this route (Ockenden 2007). It is important that Voluntary Services Managers react appropriately to legal and regulatory frameworks. In the United Kingdom these include general health and safety training, insurance cover and, sometimes, criminal record bureau checks. However, Voluntary Services Managers also have to balance risk management with risk-taking, avoiding unnecessary hurdles, and embedding equal access to volunteering opportunities. For example Sue Ryder Care in the United Kingdom has a very successful programme integrating offenders into volunteer roles in its charity shops.

Other complexities for Voluntary Services Managers range from personal issues in volunteers' lives that make it complicated for them to meet commitments, to volunteers who struggle to comply with agreed organizational protocols. However, set against these issues are the overwhelming benefits of volunteering. Volunteers remind us that care is not a commodity, a professionally delivered prescription against known problems of a 'service user'; it is a partnership that we create together as individuals, communities, and societies. It is also true that with ageing populations across the Western world, increased health-care demands and inevitable economic constraints, volunteering will become more important than ever. We need to embrace its possibilities. Voluntary Services Managers lead this ongoing quest and bear the challenge of ensuring that end-of-life care organizations do not become cosy, complacent, and inflexible about volunteer roles, but offer volunteer-centric opportunities within a culture of mutual dependence and enrichment.

I was a member of the recent U.K. Commission on the Future of Volunteering and can think of no better conclusion than to quote from its 2008 'Manifesto for Change'. 'Our vision ultimately is that volunteering becomes part of the DNA of our society—it becomes integral to the way we think of ourselves and live our lives, and we are inspired to contribute in this way. Our aim is for a culture change in society so that helping others and benefiting from a culture of mutual dependence becomes a way of life, from which the whole of society benefits.' Nowhere is this vision more pertinent than in end-of-life care and no one's role will be more significant in its delivery than that of the Voluntary Services Manager.

Barbara Monroe
St Christopher's Hospice 2009

References

Commission on the Future of Volunteering. www.volcomm.org.uk. Last accessed 6th February 2009.

Commission on the Future of Volunteering – *Manifesto for Change*. (2008). London, Volunteering England.

Field, D., Payne, S., Relf, M. and Reid, D. (2007). An overview of adult bereavement support in the United Kingdom: issues for policy and practice. *Social Science and Medicine* **64**(2), 428–438.

Help the Hospices. (2006*). Volunteer value. A pilot survey in UK hospices.* London, Help the Hospices.

Ockenden, N. (2007). *Volunteering and social policy*. London, Commission on the Future of Volunteering, Institute for Volunteering Research and Volunteering England.

Relf, M. (1998). Involving volunteers in bereavement counselling. *European Journal of Palliative Care* **5**(2), 61–65.

Rochester, C. (2006*). Making sense of volunteering; a literature review.* London, The Commission on the Future of Volunteering, Volunteering England.

Preface

Volunteers have long been an integral part of hospice and palliative care with many hospices owing their very origins to volunteers. It is reassuring that today volunteers are still central to the care and support provided by hospice services, despite the many changes and advances in hospice care and in society as a whole. Every successful team needs effective leadership, and volunteer management has evolved from an unpaid role taken on by a willing volunteer, to fast becoming a profession in its own right with competences and standards. It must, however, continue to evolve creatively if we are to meet the changing expectations of volunteers and the developing needs of the hospice and palliative care service. Hence the need for a second edition of the successful and popular first edition of this book.

This new edition brings additional chapters to set hospice volunteering in the context of the wider world of volunteering, to bring a wider international dimension to the book. These chapters give us another perspective on managing volunteers. The chapters show how similar experiences can be and that managing volunteers can be broadly the same as in the United Kingdom and that we can draw on the experience of colleagues overseas to pick up on practice and achievements. But as the chapter on community palliative care in India shows, there are radically alternative models of delivery out there that we can also admire and learn from. This second edition will also bring updated information on legal and ethical issues which face voluntary services managers today.

We hope that this book will be a useful resource to anyone involved with volunteers in hospice and palliative care and will be as valuable to those setting up new services as it will be to those with long-established volunteer teams. The book is structured in such a way that each chapter stands alone. This will allow the reader to 'dip in' for specific information or read as a whole. Chapters 1–8 focus on the context and the many facets of the role of the management of voluntary services in palliative care; Chapters 9–12 consider specific areas of volunteer involvement; and Chapters 13–16 bring an international dimension, giving us another perspective on managing volunteers. The chapters show how similar experiences can be, that managing volunteers can be broadly the same as in the United Kingdom and that we can draw on the experience of colleagues overseas to pick up on practice and achievements. But as the chapter on community palliative care in India shows, there are radically alternative models of delivery out there that we can also admire and learn from.

Whilst chapters have been cross-referenced, there may be some repetition and even some contradictions as each author describes their style and approach to the varied aspects of volunteer management. We hope that this will stimulate thought and varied ideas for your own approach to leadership and development of the volunteer programme.

We would like to thank the many contributors to this book for taking time from a busy schedule and workload to share their knowledge, expertise, and wisdom from their many and varied experiences of and observations on managing volunteers.

It is with thanks also that we recognize the help and support of Help the Hospices, AVSM (the professional association of voluntary service managers in palliative care) and Kelly Martin for her administrative support.

We would also like to thank Derek Doyle, Advisory Editor, and Georgia Pinteau, Eloise Moir-Ford, Nicola Ulyatt at OUP and Gayathri Bellan for their patience, guidance, and support.

It also seems fitting in a book about volunteer management to recognize the work of the many, many volunteers who give of their time so freely in support of hospices worldwide in so many ways. Because of their generosity of spirit, energy, and commitment, hospices are able to provide the wide range of care, services, and support that they do today.

Ros Scott
Steven Howlett
Editors
February 2009

Contents

List of contributors

Dorothy Bates
Formerly Volunteer Service Manager
St. Michael's Hospice Basingstoke
Hampshire, UK

Kathleen Defilippi
Executive Director,
South Coast Hospice,
Port Shepstone Kwa Zulu Natal,
Republic of South Africa

Dr Derek Doyle (Advisory Editor)
Founding member and international
adviser to the International Association
for Palliative and Hospice Care
(IAHPC) and Hon. Vice President of the
National Council for Palliative Care

Gill Hamilton
Formerly Volunteer Service Manager
St Columba's Hospice Edinburgh,
Scotland

Rosemary Hanley
Formerly Volunteer Service Manager
Austin and Repatriation Hospital
Heidelberg Victoria, Australia

Steven Howlett (Editor)
Senior Lecturer, School of Business and
Social Science,
Roehampton University, Roehampton

Dr Suresh Kumar
Director,
Institute of Palliative Medicine,
Calicut, Kerala, India

Silke Lean
Volunteer Service Manager,
Edenhall Marie Curie Centre Hampstead,
London, UK

Steve McCurley
US-based Consultant and Author on
Volunteer Management

Patricia McDermott
Volunteer Service Manager,
Edenhall Marie Curie Centre Hampstead,
London, UK

Mabuyi Mnguni
Deputy Director, South Coast Hospice,
Port Shepstone KwaZulu Natal,
Republic of South Africa

Suzanne O'Brien
Coordinator Hope and Cope Jewish
General Hospital Montreal,
Canada

Jenny Osterfield
Bereavement Service Co-ordinator
St Michael's Hospice Basingstoke
Hampshire, UK

Mark Restall
Independent Consultant

Ros Scott (Editor)
Director of Organizational
Development, Children's Hospice
Association Scotland, Edinburgh,
Scotland UK

Sally-Ann Spencer-Gray
Independent Consultant and Trainer

Ellen Wallace
Formerly Co-ordinator of Volunteers,
Palliative Care Service,
Royal Victoria Hospital,
Montreal, Canada

Chapter 1

Introduction

Derek Doyle

The evolution of hospice care

In many countries we have come to regard hospices as an accepted feature of our society, one that we almost take for granted, in much the same way as we expect every town to have its library, its swimming pool, and its civic centre. Most cities have at least one, its senior staff often affiliated with the local university. Most people know or have heard of someone who was cared for in a hospice. Friends and relatives are often serving as volunteers in their local hospice. Wherever we go, we see collecting cans or read of fund-raising events—all for the local hospice.

It therefore comes as a surprise to many to learn that the first 'modern' hospice only opened in 1967. The term 'modern' is used because, in the Middle Ages, there were hundreds of hospices, scattered along the trade and crusading routes of Europe, offering sustenance, care, and welcoming shelter to weary and often diseased and dying travellers. Most, if not all, were run by religious orders. Some remain to this day—wonderful museums to be visited and marvelled at with their airy rooms, drainage, and sanitation, way ahead of their time, and facilities that must have had a wonderful effect on those who sought comfort and care within their walls.

Since 1967, hospices have sprung up all over the world so that, as we write this book, there are more than 8000 hospice services worldwide. What is important, however, is the word 'services'. No longer is a hospice always a building of bricks and mortar. It is, in a sense, a philosophy of care. There may indeed be a building for inpatients but, equally, hospice care may be given in a patient's home, in the wards of a general or a specialist hospital, in a nursing or residential home, or in a day-care unit, which the patient visits from home. Indeed, as needs have been identified, it is now possible for those in prison to receive hospice care.

What is hospice care?

Whatever the place of care, the overriding needs of the patient and the underpinning principles of their care are the same. The patients are all suffering from advanced life-threatening illness. They may have only months or even weeks of life left and what they need—and what the hospice is there to provide—is relief of their suffering, whatever its cause, whatever its nature—whether it is physical, spiritual, or emotional. Hospice care focuses on quality of life rather than length of life—neither abbreviating it nor trying to extend it artificially. Not only is hospice care about quality of life—it is equally about the value of the person's life and helping him or her to find meaning in life as it draws to a close. Finally, hospice care embraces respect for the suffering and the needs of relatives and close friends.

It might well be pointed out—as indeed it has often been—that such compassionate, holistic caring is surely the hallmark of all care given to patients whatever the illness or its stage and whoever is the carer, be it doctor, nurse, pastoral care worker, or social worker. This emphasis on patient-centred care focusing on quality of life, patient autonomy, and profound respect for the individual should be an integral feature of all care. Sadly, however, that is not always the case.

In recent years, with many new techniques and drugs making cure a possibility, more effort has been spent on trying to cure than on providing care for those who cannot be cured. Increasingly, hospitals are assumed to be the best places for treatment and care when, in fact, evidence and experience show that most people with a terminal illness prefer to stay at home as long as possible, although not necessarily to die at home. Hospitals are certainly appreciated by people when they need highly specialized care, often enhanced by modern technology, but there comes a time when they want a less frenetic atmosphere, some peace and quiet to think and to enjoy time with loved ones. A hospice aims to provide that—an atmosphere tailored to the needs of the dying, a place where it is safe to laugh as well as to cry, where it is safe to 'be yourself' and, as so many people have said, a safe place to die, paradoxical as that may sound.

Why call it 'palliative care'?

In this very short space of time, the word 'hospice' has been accepted into the English language and come to mean something very special to many people. They associate it with the care their loved ones and friends received when they needed it. They know of the warmth of its care, the dedication of its staff, the visits paid to people being looked after at home, and the creative vitality of day hospices where hobbies are developed, new skills discovered, and rich friendships formed. Why then was the term 'palliative care' ever coined and adopted? What was wrong with 'hospice'?

There are several reasons. The term was probably first attached to this philosophy of care in French Canada where the word 'hospice' means something quite different from what we have been describing. There, and in many other parts of the world, it was felt that a term was needed, which described what happens in a 'hospice', a term that would be understood by doctors and nurses because it was part of their daily vocabulary. Such a word is 'palliative', which has long been used to describe comfort care when cure was impossible. Palliation might be easing pain when the underlying problem cannot be eradicated or relieving breathlessness, restoring appetite, helping sleep, or explaining what is happening to lessen the anxieties. It might simply mean being there when someone is lonely on what must surely be the loneliest journey any of us ever makes.

There is no difference between hospice and palliative care. Both describe the same thing, but whereas 'hospice' is the word beloved of the public, 'palliative care' is the term now accepted and reasonably well understood by health-care professionals the world over.

All such care must, in popular jargon, be interdisciplinary or inter-professional. This means much more than doctors, nurses, social workers, and the professions allied to medicine all working for the common good of the patient ('multiprofessional'). It means that they share a common goal for each patient under their care; that they know the skills and gifts each can bring to that care; that they share their skills and their insights so that the care they give as a team is better than could come from any one individual; and that they support each other. The analogy with a sports team is obvious—all working together, as equals, for a common goal.

When we refer to the work of the team we speak of palliative care. When we consider the role of doctors as part of that team the term palliative medicine is used, and when considering the work of the nurses, it is palliative nursing. This clearer definition of what everyone does, together with the vast increase in knowledge and expertise in recent years has brought about the recognition of both palliative medicine and palliative nursing as specialties, first in the United Kingdom and Eire, then in Australia, New Zealand, Hong Kong, Taiwan, Italy, Singapore, Romania, and Poland.

Education and training in palliative care

It has long been recognized by many health-care professionals that they need better education and training in this field of care than they ever received in the past. Who better to contribute to that than those working in palliative care, particularly when they have devoted many years to advanced training to qualify as specialists? For that reason most hospices/palliative care services have medical and nursing students to visit the units, release their senior staff to lecture in the universities and colleges of nursing, and have education departments visited by literally thousands of people each year. All of this is essential but it imposes on the staff a responsibility to see that so many professional visitors do not damage the ambience being created for the patients, or infringe their privacy and dignity.

Palliative care services

We have already seen that hospice/palliative care need not mean an inpatient unit like a mini-hospital though such units continue to be built and developed around the world. In the United Kingdom, four-fifths of them are detached from any hospital and very largely dependent on the generosity of the general public. The other one-fifth are in, or within the grounds of, National Health Service hospitals and run as part of that hospital. Busy as they always are, in fact only a small percentage of people dying with diseases, such as cancer, actually die in an inpatient palliative care unit.

Most people have their initial investigations, are diagnosed, then given their active treatment and often keep being re-admitted to general and specialist hospitals until they die. The challenge was therefore how to help them, how to offer them the highest standard of palliative care without them having to move to another place such as the district hospice/palliative care unit. The answer lay in forming hospital palliative care teams, based in secondary and tertiary referral hospitals. They could see patients with advanced illness in wards familiar to them from previous admissions, advise on appropriate care and, in so doing, enable young hospital doctors and nurses to see how effective such expert palliative care can be. Today, hospital palliative care teams are the fastest growth areas in this subject, to be found not only in every cancer centre but in many large, even world-famous hospitals in the United Kingdom, Canada, United States of America, and Australasia.

As we have said, many people when they sense or have had it confirmed that their illness is far advanced, ask to stay at home provided their loved ones, assisted by the family doctor and community nurses, will be able to look after them. To enable that to happen, community palliative care services were created and are now to be found, in their thousands, around the world. Patients are visited at home, their needs are assessed, and advice given to them, their lay carers, and to their professional carers. After that they continue to be visited, sometimes being brought in to a day hospice, sometimes helped in their visits to hospital, and sometimes offered a bed in the inpatient unit for terminal care, for control of their symptoms or as a respite for their relatives.

Most community palliative care teams are advisory as described but a few teams offer comprehensive care in the home. They take out beds, equipment, medications, carry out minor surgical procedures if they will ease the patient's suffering, and even offer round-the-clock nursing. Increasingly, as will be described in this book, they are to be found where resources are scanty, doctors and nurses are scarce, and drugs not available.

Day hospices are one of the forms palliative care can take. Patients are brought in from home by volunteer transport once or twice a week. After a cup of coffee and a chat they busy themselves with whatever activity or craft is assigned to them by the occupational therapist who has assessed their needs. It might be a long-standing hobby or interest like woodwork or painting, or a new one such as pottery, enamel work, or indoor gardening. After lunch (usually with 'just a little drink') there may be entertainment laid on, or sometimes a well-known actor or sports person may visit, until mid-afternoon when they are taken back home, usually tired but delighted to have been with others in the same boat as themselves and surprised at how much they managed to do.

Of course, not all palliative care services offer all that we have described here. Those that do, however, we might term comprehensive palliative care services. In addition to the inpatient unit with anything from 6 to more than 100 beds, there will also be a community palliative care service, a day hospice/palliative care unit, even a hospital palliative care team, a bereavement service, and an education and training programme.

Clearly, there is no right model and no wrong model. A small hospice/palliative care unit with a few beds may be exactly what a small community needs, whereas some-where else, the need is more for assistance in keeping people at home or giving respite care. What matters is that the needs of the community—be it a small town or a suburb of a major city—are thoroughly assessed before any palliative care programme is planned and then the most appropriate model established to meet those needs. Sadly, this does not always happen and, in some places, there has been over-provision of some palliative care models and even unhealthy competition between providers.

Who are the patients?

Professionals working in the field of palliative care have devised various working definitions to describe their work to the patients they are qualified to care for. Essentially, it is people with far-advanced, life-threatening illness for whom cure is not possible and for whom the focus of care must be their quality of life.

For many years, almost everyone who was referred by his/her doctor for palliative care, had a malignant disease, usually cancer. Experience had taught us that they often suffered not only appalling pain but also loss of appetite, nausea, sickness, increasing frailty, and weight loss, all of which could be helped with skilled palliation.

Gradually, it came to be recognized that the same principles could be applied to many other, non-malignant conditions, such as heart disease, respiratory problems, advanced endocrine disorders, and neurological problems, such as muscular dystrophy, motor neurone disease, and multiple sclerosis. Today, palliative care also plays a major part in the care of people with HIV and AIDS. Indeed, in several cities, special AIDS hospices have been established, and many community palliative care services are exclusively for AIDS patients.

In the adult hospices a high percentage of the patients are admitted for terminal care although, of course, they may have been under the community palliative care service for many months and also attending the day hospice. Children's hospices are different. Children are admitted for palliative respite care, emergency care, and terminal care. Most are there, as is explained in Chapter 12, to give a welcome and much-needed respite to their parents or carers and support to siblings. Many of them have very complex needs arising from congenital conditions, often quite rare, and are heavily dependent on their families to provide 24 hour care in their homes.

The workload of hospice/palliative care services

The popular image of a hospice is a place of great tranquility. People imagine staff spending most of the time sitting quietly by bedsides, admitting a new patient every few days and that few, if any, of those patients are ever able to return home but content to be there until they die.

In fact, such places are extremely busy.

The average length of time people are in a hospice/palliative care unit is usually less than two weeks. Between 40 per cent and 60 per cent are discharged home into the care of their family doctor and the community palliative care service. Most units, depending on the number of beds they have, admit between 500 and 1000 patients each year. At any one time, between 100 and 300 will be under care in their own homes. Whereas until relatively recently almost every patient had a form of cancer, today 20 per cent to 30 per cent will have some other life-threatening illness.

The professional staff

The specialist palliative care services have senior staff—physicians and nurses—who are all accredited specialists. To reach that level they have had to train for at least 8 to 10 years after qualifying as doctors or registered nurses. Supporting them are the 'professions allied to medicine' (PAMs) which include physiotherapists, occupational therapists, music and art therapists, dieticians, and nutritionists. Larger units also have at least one social worker, a pastoral care worker (chaplain), clinical pharmacist, and if they are fortunate, a clinical psychologist.

The larger hospice/palliative care units have a library with its own librarian, often serving as a resource for local universities and colleges. The educational work of the unit is led by a full-time lecturer/educationalist often assisted by other lecturers. Some of the teaching is, of course, done by other members of the clinical staff.

Supporting them all are the administrative staff under a Chief Executive responsible for the overall management, fund-raising, all staff matters, and public relations.

If there is one word which should, and indeed nearly always does, describe the work of a hospice/palliative care service, it is professionalism. Each member of staff is carefully selected, given excellent pre-service and in-service training and supervision, is well supported, and sets the highest standards for their work, their loyalty, their work relationships, whatever their role or position within the unit and its many diverse services.

The volunteers

'Professionalism' may be the word that best describes the work but ask patients and their relatives what words they would use to describe their impressions of a hospice or a palliative care unit or community service and they will say 'homely, friendly, relaxed, safe, unthreatening'. They will describe how they were always made welcome, were helped by people who were 'approachable, understanding, ready to listen, and who knew what was needed'.

There can be little doubt that hospices benefit from two very special groups—the professional staff of doctors, nurses, chaplains, and many others, who as we have seen have added to their professional training through palliative-specific training and experience. Allied to this are the many, many volunteers who give literally thousands of hours to hospices each year. Just how this army is recruited, trained, supervised, and supported, how its members are helped to work side by side with the professional team, and who leads this army—this is the content of this book.

Volunteers are so much a feature of this work that we can and do, at times, take them for granted. Not only that, we can overlook the skills needed by the person who manages the voluntary services, whether that person is termed the Volunteers Coordinator or, much more preferable, the 'Voluntary Services Manager—VSM'. This book is for them, whatever their title or job description.

Their work is difficult, always challenging, complex, varied, and often deeply rewarding. It calls for imagination and vision, infinite patience, and consummate skills of diplomacy as well as sensitive understanding of people. It calls for managerial, organizational, and leadership skills and an informed and profound understanding of hospice and palliative care, how it is provided, and who its patients and providers are.

This book has been written for them—the managers of voluntary services throughout this exciting world of hospice and palliative care.

Why this book is needed

There are many parallels between the professional ('paid') staff and the volunteers. For example, it used to be thought that any doctor or nurse could look after a person with a terminal illness—it was thought to be something that came naturally, like breathing or eating. It did not require any thought. No training was needed for it! How wrong we were. It was because of these misunderstandings that so many patients suffered as they did. Experience has shown that to do this work properly, as it deserves, and as our patients have every right to expect requires not only training, but also careful selection, inspired leadership, and understanding support. The same applies to volunteers.

Doctors and nurses need inspired, informed leadership. So do volunteers. They both need someone who understands their work, knows its challenges as well as its rewards; someone who knows how to get the best out of them and bring about genuine job satisfaction.

Professional staff need to be supported—and to feel supported—in their day-to-day work. So do volunteers. Neither group seeks sympathy or praise but they both need to know there is someone who understands how stressed they can sometimes feel, how disappointed, how frustrated.

Both professionals and volunteers like to feel that they are working in a well-organized, well-managed organization—a 'business-like one' with clear channels of communication, well-planned budgets, and well-informed senior management who appreciate what they do and who they are.

What are the key features of a voluntary services manager's job?

How curious that people ever thought anyone could manage a volunteer service. All they needed was some spare time, a charming manner, a clutch of social graces, and the gift of persuasion! Not surprisingly, experience has shown that the challenge is great and to do justice to the job it requires a special kind of person. This book looks at the work of the Manager/Coordinator of Volunteers (VSM) and sets out how to ensure that it is characterized by as high a degree of professionalism as that of any of the salaried staff.

The writer once attended a lecture about the gifts and attributes a manager of a voluntary services needed to do bring to the job. In preparation, the speaker had asked volunteers, professional staff, and even patients and relatives what they thought. She then flashed on to the screen dozens of words they had come up with—diplomacy, tact, vision, understanding of people, knowledge of palliative care, office skills, public relations skills, public speaking skills, knowledge of employment law, understanding of ethics, interviewing skills…. The list seemed endless but perhaps it was all summed up in the final quote—'She needs to be like a God but never behave like one!'

In this book, we shall address many of the responsibilities of VSMs. How do you go about recruiting and selecting, training, and supporting volunteers? How do you interview and how do you reject someone? How do you select for different roles—a vacancy in the day hospice, another one in the flower arranging team, and several in the charity shops?

What management and office skills and experience does a VSM need? Is computer literacy necessary? When does efficiency become an intrusive obsession likely to annoy the volunteers? What records are essential and what are not essential but likely to be very useful in day-to-day management?

Is it asking too much that managers have an understanding of medical ethics? As every experienced volunteer manager will attest and every long-serving hospice professional confirm, there are occasions when confidentiality is breached without people recognizing what they have done. How easy it is to tell someone of a mutual friend you saw in the hospice when doing your voluntary work there—even that is breaching confidentiality. Would an understanding of the ethics of resource allocation be helpful or an informed understanding of the issues surrounding voluntary euthanasia and physician-assisted suicide?

Are there legal issues any manager needs to be conversant with? Clearly, laws differ from one country to another, and this book has been prepared for colleagues worldwide but certain issues are shared by all. Do volunteer drivers need a special insurance policy? Who is responsible if a patient is allowed to fall out of a wheel chair being pushed by a volunteer or slips when being assisted to walk to the toilet?

This raises even bigger questions. Should volunteers ever give 'hands-on' patient care? If so, is it to save the salary of a qualified nurse or to release a nurse to do something 'more important'? Even this question leads to an even more basic one. Why do we have volunteers at all? Is it to make the place more user-friendly, more like home? Is it to save money or to do tasks modern nurses do not like doing? Is it possible to have too many volunteers around the place? Are there some tasks that volunteers should never be asked or expected to do?

As paediatricians remind us, children are not miniature adults. They differ in very many respects. Are children's hospices just adult hospices painted and equipped for little people? Could a person be equally effective and valued as a volunteer in a children's hospice as in the adult hospice down the road where they have worked for several years? This and many other issues are addressed in Chapter 12, which is devoted to children's hospices.

Are the principles and the problems the same whether you are a volunteer in a 10-bed hospice or working as part of a hospital palliative care team in a 1000-bed hospital? Are things different in Australia, North America, and India? If you are a volunteer in a deprived, AIDS-ridden part of Africa, is it reasonable that you should get some very modest payment for your work or is that changing your status from a volunteer to a member of the paid staff? This too will be addressed in the book.

Research has shown that well-trained, well-supervised volunteers are as effective at bereavement support as professional counsellors. Who is suitable for this work and how can they be trained, supervised, and supported? Should this be yet another responsibility of the VSM and if not, whose should it be?

As readers will have observed, until now we have spoken as though all volunteers are untrained people, with hearts of gold and with some time to spare to help those less fortunate than themselves. However, there are others who offer their services.

These are the highly trained health-care professionals like doctors, nurses, physiotherapists, and occupational therapists, and, an increasingly common event in modern hospice care—those who have trained in some branch of complementary or alternative medicine. What should be the relationship of the manager with them? Should they be accountable to manager or to the senior physician or director of nursing? What are the legal aspects of involving them?

No, being a manager of a voluntary service is not the easy task some people have thought it to be. We hope this book will bring clarity to it for some, will smooth the way for others, and help everyone to get even greater satisfaction out of doing it.

Chapter 2

Setting the scene: the landscape of volunteering

Steven Howlett

Introduction

This chapter focusses on the changing environment in which Voluntary Services Managers (VSM) work. The majority of the book concentrates on specific aspects of the role of the VSM looking at, among other things, their place in the organizational structure of hospices, the skills and techniques they need to manage volunteers appropriately and effectively, and ethical issues that they may encounter. We must realize, however, that how we manage volunteers within the hospice walls is impacted upon by the world outside, and that world is changing. But how is it changing? What are the trends that may effect what VSMs do? Are the same sorts of people volunteering for the same sorts of reasons? Is government interest in volunteering encouraging more people to volunteer, or is the push to give voluntary organizations a greater role in public services merely making more organizations compete for the same volunteers? This chapter will look at recent trends, try to highlight which remain pretty much constant, and which are changing and how. Through this, the chapter poses some questions that readers may want to consider as they work through the remainder of the book.

Volunteers for health-related matters

The importance of volunteering hardly needs to be stressed to anyone reading this book. While it is helpful to acknowledge that volunteering has been an innate part of societies throughout history, it is more helpful perhaps to reflect on volunteering and its importance in health and social care in more recent times.

Surveys suggest that volunteering in this field has always been popular—and continues to be. Despite the development of the welfare state in the 1940s, which some predicted would undermine the need for volunteering, the involvement of volunteers within health and social care and the wider social services remained strong. It was also the area that awoke government interest in the potential of volunteering in the 1960s, and helped set the framework for how volunteers are supported and managed today. The first volunteer manager in the United Kingdom, for example, was in health when Fulton Hospital created a manager role in 1963. Elements of the volunteer-supporting infrastructure, that we are familiar with today, has its roots in managing volunteers within the caring sector in this era. The Volunteer Centre UK (now Volunteering England) had its genesis in a recommendation by the Aves Committee, which was set up to look at volunteering in social services. Although the remit of the committee concentrated on volunteers in statutory services, it was interested in searching for distinctions between the role of paid staff and volunteers. It also recognized that the need to professionalize services must include training volunteers received but this should not erode the difference between paid and unpaid staff[1]. These are important issues and represent something of the continuity of the landscape, resolving, or at least managing these issues remains a task of VSMs. We will return to this in the following paragraphs. First let us consider one very important trend—are volunteer numbers rising or falling?

How many people volunteer?

Can we expect that the field of health and social care will continue to remain important and attract enough people to volunteer? And how does this translate to the hospice movement? At the outset, it is worth noting what we know about the total numbers of volunteers. So often we hear stories of a decline in civic attitudes and of less people willing to get involved. But behind the headlines the picture depends on what we are looking at. In England, for example, a survey in 2007–2008 found that 43 per cent of the adult population had volunteered formally at least once over the previous 12 months. Although data is not available to compare over the longer term with confidence we can, at least, compare the most recent figurers against 2001. Overall, this suggests levels of volunteering in 2007 were the same as they were in 2001 (73 per cent and 74 per cent, respectively). But we should note these impressive figures include formal and informal volunteering (i.e. formal volunteering is within an organization, while informal volunteering is more akin to neighbourliness or doing favours for others). In fact, levels of formal volunteering have risen from 39 to 43 per cent over the period and it is informal volunteering that has dipped[2]. In Scotland, however, the picture is slightly different. Figures there show a fall from 43 per cent in 2004 to 38 per cent in 2005 and then to 32 per cent in 2006. In Northern Ireland there is a similar story, a 2007 survey shows levels of volunteering in Northern Ireland at 21 per cent down from 29 per cent in 2001[3].

The overall pool of volunteers from where hospices might draw seems therefore to vary from place to place in the United Kingdom, and it is not always clear whether the pool is expanding or contracting. We could say though that it remains relatively healthy even if it is not expanding at the rate some might expect, given the attention volunteering has received from policy makers[4].

What we know about who volunteers

Unfortunately, it isn't possible to drill down further into these existing surveys to get an idea of trends in volunteering within hospices. We can get a very general picture from national surveys, for example, we know from one survey that 18 per cent of all volunteers in England are involved in the field of 'health and disability'. This certainly stands up well against other fields—just two areas, 'Education' (22 per cent) and

'Religion' (14 per cent) claim a greater share of volunteer involvement with volunteering in sports having the same share as health and disability[5]. As far as we can compare with past surveys this remains fairly constant, although there are always issues with time series in volunteering because very few surveys are conducted holding important methodological factors constant, including asking the same questions with the same amount of prompting and with the same sample sizes. How far does this help us? Identifying volunteers in health and disability can only be a rough proxy—it is not the same as hospice involvement. Furthermore, when volunteers are surveyed they can choose to identify their volunteering as to do with 'children' or 'the elderly'—both of which are categories appearing in the survey. In either case, of course, volunteering for children or the elderly could be in a hospice setting.

It would be helpful to have more specific data on hospice volunteers. But even this would only help if we had a time series from which we could gauge whether hospices were attracting sufficient numbers of volunteers. We do not have this and neither do we have data on the profile of volunteers in hospices. That is, we do not know whether more of older or younger people volunteer, or whether volunteers are a good reflection of the communities in which hospices sit. Although when Chapter 7 in this book talks about most volunteers starting their volunteering when they are middle aged, this may be a picture many VSMs recognize and it does accord with what we know about volunteers in general.

Do other trends in hospices accord with what we know about general trends in volunteering? Next we consider general trends from which VSMs can start to draw their own conclusions about how their hospices perform.

Gender

Most people when asked, assume more women than men volunteer. And while this is supported by survey data, again it depends what aspect of volunteering we are asking about. We see, for example, that 29 per cent of women volunteered regularly in 2007–2008 compared to 25 per cent of men[6], but if we look at different roles and activities, men volunteer more than women for some of them. Importantly, for this book, we can say from surveys that women in England are more likely than men to volunteer in health/disability organizations. To find more men than women represented as volunteers we would need to look in sports organizations[7].

Age

When looking at the ages of volunteers we see that most volunteering is done in the 'middle years'. That is, the youngest and oldest age groups volunteer less[7]. VSMs will of course know their own volunteer profile, but when they are looking to recruit, it is useful to know that this pattern does not seem to change much over time.

Ethnic origin

However, when we consider patterns of volunteering by different ethnic origins, recent surveys paint a different picture to earlier surveys. This may be because our knowledge has increased as more surveys have been conducted. For some time it was believed that Black and minority ethnic volunteers were well represented in their own communities and largely engaged within informal volunteering. However, more recent surveys in England and Scotland show that people from non-white backgrounds have been found to be equally likely to be involved in regular, formal volunteering as their white counterparts. There are some variations, the term black and minority ethnic itself covers a range of communities, and if we examine survey data more closely, we find that Asian and Chinese people were found to be less likely to be regular formal volunteers in surveys in England. Even then there are further differences; for example, for people with an Asian background, it was found 22 per cent of people with an Indian background, 16 per cent of Pakistani people, and 15 per cent of Bangladeshi people volunteered[7].

Employment, education and socioeconomic status

Surveys have also shown that employment status and education level is a strong indicator of the likelihood of people volunteering. One of the barriers mentioned most frequently by people when asked about volunteering is a lack of time; so contrary perhaps to what might seem to be common sense, the unemployed are less likely to volunteer than those who are working. Among the employed, those in full-time employment volunteer less than people who are employed part time or the self-employed.

Surveys also consistently show that people with a higher socioeconomic status (e.g. those in higher managerial or professional occupations) are more likely to volunteer than people in manual jobs. The same is true for higher qualifications—the more qualifications someone has, the more likely they are to volunteer. For example, those with a degree or above are two-and-a-half times more likely to volunteer than those with no qualifications.

Although it is difficult to make accurate comparisons over time, it does seem that there is a lot of continuity about who volunteers. Where we see change—for example, when we look at the ethnic background of volunteers—it could be, as suggested, we know more now and are able to see the picture more clearly. What this means for a VSM is that the pool from which volunteers are drawn is relatively stable. And while again, on the one hand this is comforting; on the other there has been a lot of work in recent times not least by government to try to increase this pool, which seems to have had limited impact.

Trends inside and outside the hospice

We now turn from looking at trends in numbers to look at some key issues that are impacting on volunteering, and we will focus on a selection of trends that will frame how we look at the rest of this book. First we look at diversity. Diversity is an area in which there is broad agreement—it is good to diversify volunteers and we will consider how diversity has been encouraged and facilitated but also why barriers continue to exist for some volunteers. Then we consider the motivations of volunteers to see if there are any trends to note here. These, in turn, will highlight some of the trends about who volunteers and raise questions about how we manage volunteers.

The important issue here is the extent to which volunteering is becoming more formalized, and we will consider the drivers for this, and the pros and cons of a more formalized approach to volunteer management. Finally, we will look at how government interest in volunteering has changed over time. This will allow us to draw together the issues explored in this chapter.

Diversity

We live in an increasingly diverse society, and one in which we recognize that people have a right to be involved in, and to be able to give their time freely, to organizations that recruit volunteers. Added to this is the gradual breaking down of the image of volunteering as an exclusive pastime—something only practised by a select section of the community. Diversity within volunteering is also receiving a stimulus through government policy objectives. Public Service Agreement (PS4), has since 2004 been focussed on increasing volunteering from groups at risk of social exclusion (and initiatives such as 'Goldstar' and 'Volunteering for All' have been part of this). In short, the environment in which volunteer-involving organizations operate has changed when it comes to diversity.

The Compact's Volunteering Code of Good Practice for England also identifies the importance of tackling any discrimination to ensure that volunteering is open to all[8]. This may include, but is not restricted to overt discrimination. One study by the Institute for Volunteering Research, for example, looked at the barriers facing potential volunteers and identified a set of 'psychological barriers', which included time, the image volunteering has among non-volunteers, the self-image of people at risk of exclusion, and concerns about losing benefits. Potential volunteers had exaggerated ideas of what their time commitment would need to be in order to participate as volunteers; they also had stereotypical ideas of who volunteered and what they did. Allied to this they had self-image concerns, which manifested itself as a lack of confidence that they would fit with what organization wanted from their volunteers. And, often, people in the study who received benefits worried about losing them if they volunteered. The study found a whole host of physical barriers too, for example, not knowing how to get involved, opportunities that just did not appeal, and opportunities that were physically inaccessible for them.

There are persuasive arguments for increasing diversity, namely, that by making organizations inclusive they can address and overcome systems and procedures that may be discriminatory; that diversity draws in a wider and more varied pool of skills and experience, and that diverse volunteers reflect *and* cater for diverse local communities and client groups. And of course, it will enlarge the pool of potential volunteers. Looking across the literature on barriers and diversity, the emerging picture is of a range of issues that are far from insurmountable. We need to ask ourselves therefore; when we look at the trends of who volunteers—are the people who volunteer more the ones who are able to overcome barriers better? Who have the confidence in their own skills and abilities; the networks to get involved or ability to access existing volunteering infrastructure and the ability to overcome access issues—whether that be the transport to get to opportunities or access to alternative care for children or relatives that means they have the time to volunteer? In other words, if we want to see more volunteers from other sections of society, can we address barriers and help make it happen?

Motivations

Do motivations change over time and, therefore, should they be considered in this chapter? One theme we can identify and consider is whether motivations are changing in the sense that people appear to be keener to get something from their volunteering. This may not be because motivations are changing *per se* and people are developing more instrumental motives at the expense of altruistic motivations. What we identify as people expressing motivations in terms of what they can get from volunteering may just be an indication of the successful promotion of volunteering as a reciprocal relationship. There is a well-known piece of research[9], which tries to identify what volunteering is by presenting a variety of volunteer roles to a group of people and asking them to identify which are done by volunteers. The results show that people are more likely to identify a role as a volunteer-one if they feel the person gets less out of the role than they put in. But times change and many organizations realize that if they are to attract volunteers they must offer something to volunteers. Without the lure of pay, this 'something' is a chance for volunteers to answer the needs and wants that attract them to volunteer in the first place. In other words organizations need to answer people's motivations.

This begs some interesting questions—can we identify motivations and, if so, how do we respond to them?

The area of volunteer motivations is complex and it is often said that there are as many motivations to volunteer as there are volunteers. One line of research suggests that motivations can be categorized into six areas covering things like, the wish to acquire new skills or use existing experience; to help get over some trauma of their own; or to meet and socialize with like-minded people[10]. Another set of literature looks at motivations in terms of how volunteers express their own goals, and this is often in terms of learning new skills, but frequently it is also in terms of 'giving something back'. Practically, VSMs can use this information, and we highlight a couple of findings from the literature that illustrate how research into motivations may be used. The first is that volunteers can be attracted by literature that appeals to their reason for volunteering. So, if someone is inclined to volunteer to meet their need to express their own values, recruitment literature written in these terms will appeal to those people[11]. So far so good. But, we are also conscious that volunteers do not always know what is motivating them, making the VSMs' task of identifying and then responding to those motives all the more difficult. Here again, analysing trends helps us; broadly speaking, younger people are more likely to be looking for experience, and older people want to volunteer to contribute to the community.

VSMs should be aware of another factor muddying how we might use this information. Motivations change as volunteers spend time in organizations, so what is identified as a motivation at the interview stage might have changed 6 months or a year down the line—another reason to have regular meetings with them. Although, inevitably the picture is complex, one identifiable general trend is for older volunteers to come to value the social aspect of their volunteering over and above other motives.

In other words, whatever motivated your volunteers to start, and however you identified ways to meet that motivation, the chances are that after a while your volunteers will value what you do to support the social aspects of their volunteering and it may well be this that is keeping them in your organization.

The formalization of volunteering

A key trend—and challenge—for volunteering is the degree to which it is becoming more formalized. Volunteering it is argued, is a diverse phenomenon in which people get involved in all manner of activities in all manner of organizations. Corresponding to this diversity of volunteering we might expect an equally diverse range of management ideas. But we are seeing the expansion of 'the workplace model', in which volunteering looks like paid work, but without the pay[12]. The reasons for this can be found in the environment in which volunteering works—the encouragement by statutory authorities to deliver public services funded by public money, which, in turn, demands adherence to policies and procedures while working to contracted outcomes means volunteers are more tightly managed to achieve those ends. Another trend ratcheting up formalization is risk and the fear of litigation in which organizations fear being exposed to risk through not to having adequate management systems—something Chapter 8 explains well.

But, volunteer managers face a conundrum. On the one hand volunteers tell us that what they want from their volunteering is fun and they tell us that they are put off by too much bureaucracy. On the other hand they tell us that while they want a light touch, they also want to know that their volunteering is well organized. Kathy Gaskin's instructive and practical research says it all in the title— volunteers want 'a choice blend'[13]. We must add to this the trends we noted earlier—some sections of the community are put off by bureaucracy and procedures and so management can act against diversity. What may seem good practice to a hospice and to the VSM—interviewing volunteers, for example, may be the thing that puts people off applying. What is the point of encouraging people to volunteer as a step towards paid work, for example, if the first thing they meet is an interview—the world of paid work replicated in the world of volunteering?

Yet, many VSMs, and some of those appearing in this volume, argue that such systems are necessary. In highly regulated environments such as a hospice, they may be necessary. Hospices are scrutinized by a range of regulatory bodies—Care Commission, NQuiz, Environmental Health, HSE, Charity regulators—to name just a few. But VSMs need to look for appropriate management too— for example, do shop volunteers need the same sort of management as volunteers working directly with patients? VSMs have a fine line to walk and need to balance management approaches with the need to recruit and retain volunteers; if retired people are being recruited as volunteers, is a replica of the world of work what they want? When looking at diversifying volunteers, are procedures a barrier; what role do VSMs have in protecting the diversity not of volunteers, but of volunteering? None of this is to say that volunteer management is at odds with how volunteers want to be managed, but the move towards formalization and what volunteers want from their involvement needs skilled balancing from skilled managers.

Government influence

Finally, underpinning much of what has been said earlier is the influence of government. This is having a profound effect in changing the environment in which VSMs work. We are living at a time when government has never been more interested in encouraging more people to volunteer. Barbara Monroe notes in the preface that she was a member of the recent U.K. Commission on the Future of Volunteering, which articulated that volunteering should become part of the DNA of society. The Commission was chaired by Dame Julia Neuberger who was subsequently appointed to advise the Prime Minister on volunteering matters. Dame Neuberger is a supporter of the idea of volunteer management and has voiced her idea that chief executives of volunteer-involving organizations ought to have some experience as a volunteer manager. Such untrammelled support is astonishing when we consider how far volunteering has come in the last 15 years—from something spoken about usually in connection to voluntary organizations to an important policy aim. Volunteering carries the hopes of adding significantly to the delivery of public services and to underpinning a collective sense of citizenship as well as expressing what it means to be a part of a community. It has attracted considerable resources because of this, but at the time of writing, wider economic conditions mean that this level of funding may not continue. This makes it even more important to note that the resources that have been put into volunteering have been skewed. They have been aimed at younger people, with an ultimate aim of helping them into paid work and learning how to be responsible citizens. They have also been skewed towards encouraging people at risk of social exclusion to be involved in communities, and towards 'capacity building' of organizations to involve more people under-represented as volunteers or to deliver public services. In other words, these resources have not necessarily been focussed on managing the solid body of existing volunteers. At the same time, the models of volunteer management are being squeezed and shaped into an ever smaller number of templates. The dominance of the formal model risks curtailing the initiative of VSMs in favour of policies, procedures, and rules. Whether this is something to be embraced or resisted is not for this chapter to say, but without recognizing the environment in which we work, it is easy to have our heads down with busy work loads and then look up one day to find the world has changed.

Conclusion

This chapter offers a brief overview of current trends and issues in volunteer management. Outside of the hospice the volunteer environment is changing and it will continue to impact on VSMs. Some things are not changing much—we are broadly seeing the same number of people volunteering in the same areas. But other things are changing and some are changing rapidly; volunteers it seems are getting more demanding, they want organizations to be able to show them why they should give their time to that organization. Some volunteers are also increasingly interested in short-term high-impact volunteering opportunities rather than the longer-term volunteering commitments upon which so many hospice services depend.

One of the key changes we are seeing is the expansion of volunteer management, but along the route of formal practices akin to managing paid staff. But volunteering is different. Often, volunteering takes place within structured and seemingly bureau-cratic organizations. Volunteering, however, is not paid work and it retains something of the value of collective action, of the pooling of time and effort to address need. This does need a different management approach—or at least recognition of how and when to apply the techniques of management. Most of the rest of the chapters in this volume address managing volunteers in hospices from this view point. It is hoped that this chapter has also added some context so that VSMs can also question as they read. VSMs can learn from the following chapters, from experienced managers who have much to teach. There are also alternative models and the chapters outlining how colleagues in other countries go about their tasks also show us that we must keep questioning how we work if we are to continue to be creative and innovative in the development and management of voluntary services in an ever-changing and developing society.

References

1 Davis Smith, J. (1996). 'Should Volunteers be Managed?' In *Voluntary Agencies: Challenges of Organisation and Management* (eds. D. Billis and M. Harris). Basingstoke, Macmillan.

2 Low, N. S., Butt, A., Ellis Paine, and Davis Smith J. (2007). *Helping Out: A National Survey of Volunteering and Charitable Giving.* London, Cabinet Office.

3 Rochester, C. A., Ellis Paine, and Howlett, S. (2009). *Volunteering in the 21st Century.* Basingstoke, Palgrave.

4 Who *Volunteers? Volunteering Trends: 2000-2007 A Briefing from nfpSynergy* Available online at http://www.nfpsynergy.net/includes/documents/cm_docs/2008/v/volunteeringtrendsjan08.pdf

5 Low, N. S., Butt, A., Ellis Paine, and Davis Smith, J. (2007). *Helping Out: A National Survey of Volunteering and Charitable Giving.* London, Cabinet Office.

6 Communities and Local Government. (2008). Citizenship Survey: 2007–08 (April 2007 – March 2008), England & Wales: Cohesion research statistical release 4, London, CLG.

7 Rochester, C. A., Ellis Paine, and Howlett, S. (2009). *op cit.*

8 Commission for the Compact. (2005). *Volunteering Compact Code of Good Practice.* Birmingham, Commission for the Compact.

9 Cnaan, R., Handy, F., and Wadsworth, M. (1996). Defining who is a Volunteer: Conceptual and empirical considerations. *Nonprofit and Voluntary Sector Quarterly* 25, 364–383.

10 Clary, E., Snyder, M., and Ridge, R. (1992). 'Volunteers' Motivations: A functional strategy for the recruitment, placement and retention of volunteers' *Nonprofit Management and Leadership* 2, 333–350.

11 Clary, E., Snyder, M., and Ridge, R. (1992). *op cit.*

12 Rochester, C. (2006). *Making Sense of Volunteering. A Literature Review.* London, Volunteering England for The Commission on the Future of Volunteering.

13 Gaskin, K. (2003). *A Choice Blend: What Volunteers Want from Organisation and Management*, London, Institute for Volunteering Research.

Chapter 3

The management role of the Voluntary Services Manager

Dorothy Bates

There are a number of titles applied to the person who managers volunteers in a hospice, in recent times the most frequently used has been 'Volunteer Coordinator'. All are required to act as managers and are increasingly recognized and known as Voluntary Services Managers (VSM)[1]. There is however, some debate about the relevant models of management appropriate for working with volunteers. The conclusion is perhaps not so much that one model is more appropriate than another but more about finding a management style 'in keeping with the values and ethos of voluntary action'[2].

This chapter sets out to explain the diverse role of the VSM, promoting the idea that the person appointed to such a post, in whatever size of organization, should have the experience and calibre to reflect the responsibilities involved. Organizations do not always recognize the skills required and some assume that to 'organize' volunteers, who are freely giving of their time, it is easier than managing staff. In so doing, organizations can enter in to a circle of ineffectuality, often resulting in unhappy and unproductive volunteers and a negative approach throughout the organization to the benefits of working with volunteers and volunteer management.

So, what is it about the role that moves it from a coordinating role to one of management?

First, coordinating is one-dimensional, implying the organization of a group of like-minded individuals who all agree on a common task and the way to carry out that task. In hospices, volunteers, if managed effectively, can provide a vibrant, energized, and focussed workforce, capable of contributing to and enhancing the quality of the care provided, whilst also allowing the budget to be extended in imaginative and creative ways. Such a workforce is made up of a complex and diverse group of people. Diversity of people and tasks requires careful management.

Volunteers can be found in all sorts of organizations, some are 'staffed' entirely by volunteers, while some have a mix of volunteers and paid staff. Hospices and other palliative care organizations are in the latter category with the core of the service provided by paid staff. While volunteers often outnumber the staff (and, in some cases, might even be seen as a threat to paid staff), staff and volunteers are required to work alongside and support each other in what is often a fragile and highly charged atmosphere. It falls to the VSM to be responsible for good volunteer/staff relations and to facilitate an effective working relationship— a complex task!

The tasks and responsibilities carried out by volunteers do not exist in isolation to the work of the organization. The scope and volume of these volunteer activities will vary depending on the organization's willingness to harness these skills together with the success and development of the organization itself. In some organizations, however, the significant contribution of volunteers will also shape the organization.

Organizations, when planning future strategy, must consider any volunteer contribution anticipated alongside resultant resource implications. For example, in most day-care services, volunteers play a large part, whether it is to drive, to offer diversional therapy, to make teas/coffees, etc. In planning to introduce or expand a day-care service, it makes sense that the provider of these resources, the VSM, is involved at the strategic and early planning stages of such a project. Availability (or otherwise) of possible volunteers, training, and support costs, all need to be taken into account but are frequently overlooked at the initial planning stage. Volunteers are not stored in cupboards waiting to be produced whenever needed at a moments notice—a frequent misapprehension amongst paid staff!

Finally, in acknowledging that it is the VSM's responsibility to provide the equivalent of the 'human resources' function in recruiting, selecting, training, and supporting the organization's volunteers, then it is beyond doubt that it is indeed a complex management role, ideally part of the Senior Management Team.

Before examining this role in greater detail, it is important to clarify one other, often misunderstood, dimension. The role cannot be to manage the volunteer work force per se, for it is widely accepted that no manager can effectively manage large numbers of people. Since many hospice volunteer programmes number in the hundreds, clearly this would be an impossible task. And so it is the voluntary service that is managed, while the direction of the volunteers themselves is devolved to department managers/ team leaders just as in the case of paid staff.

In summary, the major role of the VSM is in strategic planning with senior managers, recruitment selection and deployment of volunteers, and working with individual staff to help them effectively manage, train, and retain their volunteers.

Working in palliative care

Many of the fundamental aspects of volunteer management in palliative care are the same as in any other organization but there are some specific elements that are important and which influence both the job content and the person specification for the role incumbent.

Working in an environment where people die has a high emotional content, which means that much more care is required in the recruitment, selection, training, and support of volunteers.

It is vitally important that the VSM is personally emotionally strong and able to understand and support volunteers exposed to the sadness of loss and bereavement.

VSMs should have a firm grasp of the philosophy underpinning the care given whether or not they themselves are from a health-care background. In many hospices, the VSM attends the weekly multidisciplinary review of patient care giving them a regular background and insight as well as contributing to discussions and planning for patients.

The management role

Planning for volunteers

In planning for a voluntary service the first task is to help the organization to focus on how it intends to relate to volunteers. The following fundamental questions must be considered and agreed:

+ Why does the organization wish to involve volunteers? (Is it just because most other units have them or, as it needs to be, from a genuine belief that volunteers will truly bring benefits?)

+ What are the organization's expectations of volunteers?

+ Will the organization be prepared actively and openly to embrace the involvement of volunteers throughout the organization and to promote this among the staff?

+ What resources is the organization prepared to devote to the development of a voluntary service?

Once these general principles have been agreed by the Board of Trustees and Senior Management Team, there is in place a firm foundation on which to build a successful voluntary service. Everyone in the organization then knows what to expect and what is expected of them and it is a powerful motivating force for volunteers, encouraging loyalty and commitment.

A similar exercise should be undertaken to define the aim and establish principles to underpin the work of the voluntary services department itself. For example, an agreed aim might read:

'… to provide voluntary support for the organization, to contribute to the improved quality of life of patients and their carers, whilst enabling volunteers to achieve their individual potential and maximum satisfaction'.[3]

Principal functions of the department might include[3]:

+ Recruiting, selecting, and placing suitable volunteers who will:
  - Provide to patients and carers a service that complements that which is provided by the professional team, and
  - Support other staff in the performance of their duties.

+ Develop and implement policy and best practice in the day-to-day deployment of volunteers.

+ Develop the potential of the volunteer resource and encourage new initiatives to meet identified needs.

+ Monitor and evaluate services to maximize their effectiveness and improve practice.

More detailed decisions on where volunteers work, what they do, and how they do it become part of the ongoing management role of the VSM. These decisions should all be based on written policies and procedures, covering areas such as administrative and clinical procedures, strategies, and statistics, and review processes[3].

Strategic planning

As the organization develops and external circumstances change so is vital that the VSM keeps abreast about the changing needs of both the organization and the wider world of palliative care. In order to support and contribute to the strategic and business planning of the organization, the VSM must maintain an awareness of wider external implications for volunteering as outlined in Chapter 2. This includes such issues as the changing political climate, including government activities, policies and new legislation, changing demographic trends, including an understanding of the local cultural environment where attitudes towards volunteering may be different, and the changing economic climate. Assuming that hospices continue to depend on a significant contribution from volunteers, the trends in availability of volunteers as a resource must be a key consideration in the planning process.

Budgeting for volunteers

Establishing and managing a realistic budget, operating within it, and reviewing performance before re-negotiating a new budget creates an efficient and effective way to develop the volunteer service in line with the organization's working principles and priorities.

Assessing costs

Some organizations make a mistake by believing that the introduction of volunteers is a cheap option, with such low costs, that no formal budgeting is necessary. It becomes clear how necessary it is to agree to a budget, allocate resources, and effectively manage them by examining some of the possible costs of a voluntary service:

◆ Good volunteer practice in the United Kingdom[4], based on equality of opportunity for all, encourages the reimbursement of expenses to all volunteers.

◆ Recruitment resources such as advertising, leaflets, etc.

◆ Training and support for volunteers using facilitators, rooms, equipment, etc.

◆ Salary costs for the VSM together with their ongoing training and support.

◆ Training and support for staff in working with volunteers

◆ Insurance cover for the work of the volunteers.

◆ Other overhead costs. (The element often forgotten in the planning for volunteers is the allocation of such simple resources as—where will the person sit or will there be a spare computer available during the time the volunteer is on duty?)

A detailed costing exercise is thus the first important step of budget planning. The VSM will then discuss with the line manager (or Chief Executive, depending on the size of the organization) the allocation of appropriate resources.

Allocation of resources

The allocation of resources to the volunteer department should be no different than for any other department in the organization. It may be that all staff in small embryonic units combine forces to raise funds to obtain the wherewithal to operate. However, in larger and more established organizations, funding needs to be organized through a central source, not only to achieve control and consistency of resource allocation, but also to avoid duplication of fund-raising activity and running the risk of creating fund-raising fatigue amongst possible donors. In any case, funding will probably come from a number of different sources and this income should form the basis of resources available to meet the organization's expenditure needs.

Budget setting

The agreed budget is usually set in advance on an annual basis with reviews carried out regularly during that time to monitor effectiveness and to allow the readjustment of targets where this is possible. Most organizations will have their own timing and procedures for the management of budgets and so naturally the process for the volunteer department will form part of these. A VSM looking to acquire the appropriate knowledge base to participate in budget setting, should find it as part of any basic diploma-type management course, or as the basis for short one-off courses often run by local or national training agencies.

The human resources manager

Although managing volunteers does have specific professional standards of its own there are certain principles of human resources management, which serve the volunteer world well and require key skills from a VSM. In particular, this is the case in small organizations where no one specializes in the HR function.

Recruitment and selection

Recruitment and selection is discussed in detail in Chapter 5; however, it is worth considering, in this context, the skills required by the VSM. Clearly, the VSM with no previous experience needs to acquire knowledge and confidence in interviewing skills and should have access to a private room in which to meet potential volunteers.

One of the most difficult situations to handle in the selection process is 'saying no'. Palliative care it is sometimes not the right environment, and so an offer of time and skills has to be turned down. Although it is occasionally possible to guide potential volunteers in another direction, it requires skilled handling on the part of the VSM to minimize the disappointment for the volunteer and at the same time to protect the reputation of the organization.

Training and support

An overview of skills relating to training and support are outlined in the following paragraphs; however, each is addressed in more depth in Chapters 6 and 7.

Assessing training and support needs of volunteers and identifying how to meet them is done by the VSM in conjunction with each department concerned. A knowledge and understanding of this process is a key skill for a VSM to have or to acquire.

Although most training sessions will involve members of the professional team, some sessions, such as introducing new volunteers to the organization's policies and procedures, can be led by the skilled VSM. As well as being able to lead a training session, it is important that the VSM is at ease in facilitating groups since regular meetings of volunteer teams is a common way to offer ongoing regular support, an opportunity to address any issues of concern, and to communicate information about organization developments and events.

Volunteers who are distressed or upset by their work for any reason need to know they can go to the VSM for support, particularly if they feel unable to talk to anyone else in the organization. The VSM needs to be familiar with basic counselling skills and be a good listener.

Motivation, retention, and guidance

Hospices and other palliative care organizations are likely to attract a significant number of volunteers in the first instance because of their belief in and support for the cause itself. At this point, understanding what brings someone to volunteer is a key aspect of the selection process as it may determine whether or not you, as the VSM, decide to accept this offer of help.

Since introducing a new volunteer to the organization and providing training is a fairly long process with a significant investment of time and resources, it becomes important to encourage good volunteers to stay. In the United Kingdom, increasing competition for people prepared to volunteer is another factor making it important to retain the volunteers already in place[4]. Although the research evidence for what measures can be put in place to help retain volunteers is inconclusive, several studies have shown that volunteers want their motivations addressed and to be and effectively supported.

One of the findings of a survey, which produced other interesting conclusions about what volunteers look for from the hospices in which they work stated: 'In order to retain support—both as fund-raisers and as volunteers—hospices must ensure that volunteers are involved, understand, and agree with the working practice of voluntary hospices'[5]. A different survey reports: 'There is some evidence that the introduction of changes without consultation or discussion with volunteers may have had a negative effect upon the commitment, sense of belonging, and motivation of some long-serving volunteers'[6].

Ongoing training provides an opportunity to show that the organization values the work of the volunteers, and the regular support of team meetings offers the chance to discuss issues of concern.

The role of the VSM here is not an easy one. Volunteers often feel very strongly about certain issues, sometimes with justification, sometimes not. For the VSM, deciding what to take further and what to challenge comes from knowing the organization, its people, its policies and procedures, and priorities. Volunteers need to trust the VSM and understand that their point of view will be heard and respected even if, in the end, it is impossible to meet their request. The ability to handle difficult situations is vital.

There are many other examples of difficult situations which a VSM must be skilled enough to handle. It may be from a volunteer becoming too old or unable to carry out duties safely to volunteers who continually overstep boundaries, from a volunteer suffering a personal bereavement to a conflict of opinion whether with staff or other volunteers. Negotiating between volunteers and staff requires significant diplomacy and tact. The VSM must be readily accessible to both volunteers and staff in an effort to keep a finger 'on the pulse' and to address difficult situations before the need arises to resort to formal procedures.

There is some debate about whether the principles of appraisal and review could or should be applied to volunteers. Whilst acknowledging that some volunteers (e.g. those gaining experience for a future career) might welcome an in-depth appraisal with targets and learning objectives, it is important to remember that many volunteers do not want to be involved in such serious undertakings. This is a good example of the need to balance the good intention of the willing citizen with the developing professionalism of the world of volunteering. Volunteers, however, do like to know if they are doing a good job or if they can do better. Consequently, feedback is important. Taking time with a volunteer to look at their contribution to the organization is a way of valuing them and can do much to both motivate and encourage a high quality of 'performance'. This is most effectively carried out by the leader of the team in which the volunteer works. The role of the VSM is to work with the team leader in setting up these meetings, supporting the team leader in carrying them out, and monitoring the outcomes.

There is little doubt that the subject of motivation is complex, but it is an area where the VSM must have insight and knowledge if valued volunteers are to be encouraged to want to stay.

Regulations

People volunteer for many reasons and, for most, there is an element of altruism and citizenship involved. For some, their wish is 'to serve'; for others, they strive to 'make a difference', both groups often driven by an idealistic zeal! It is easy, under these circumstances, for staff in organizations to overlook, and hard for some volunteers to accept, that not 'anything goes', and activities can be restricted by the bounds of the laws of the land. The VSM's role is not only to ensure that good practice is followed, but also a greater challenge is often in enabling the enthusiastic volunteer to understand the need to comply with the regulations.

Since it is normal practice for all volunteers to be covered by the organization's insurance policies, it is an important task for the VSM to ensure clarity of volunteer role definition as demanded by insurance companies, taking in to account a risk assessment of tasks to be undertaken.

Staff and volunteers working together

Paid staff can often feel threatened by the introduction of volunteers[7]. In order to help maximize the mutual benefits, it is an important responsibility of the VSM to reassure staff about the place in the organization of the volunteers by providing a framework where the role and status is defined and understood. This could be presented visually by including the volunteer roles in the organization chart. In addition, staff job descriptions should include a paragraph on their responsibility towards volunteers.

When introducing a new volunteer project, the VSM can gain the confidence of staff members by involving them at every step of the way from the planning stage onwards.

This approach has the advantage of encouraging staff to 'own' the project and to support it even through difficult times. In addition, asking team members to participate in the training of volunteers often eases their anxieties about how a project will work and the part the volunteers will play. It also gives an opportunity to the volunteers to explore their thoughts and ideas with the staff thus engendering an atmosphere of trust. However, while it is important that the VSM reinforces the positive message about working with volunteers, they must also be open and willing to hear any voices of concern, and work towards resolving any problems from any source.

Once volunteers are in place, it is important to maintain liaison with the department staff and review how the volunteer role is progressing as well as keeping lines of communication open with the volunteers. It should be clear to whom the volunteers are accountable and to whom they should go if there is a problem. The role of the VSM is to offer individual support to this member of staff and, in addition, may also provide written guidelines or training if it is felt necessary. Volunteers value feedback, and the person in the role of supervisor should be helped to perform this role with each volunteer.

Often, the sheer numbers of volunteers working in a department together with frequent shift variations for staff make communication and supervision difficult. At the very least, there should be regular volunteer team meetings at which a member of the staff team is present. It may be appropriate to appoint key members of staff and/or volunteer team leaders to represent the views of both groups and thus develop a sharing of ideas and views.

Volunteer team leaders can also undertake other key roles and this concept is particularly beneficial in large organizations where often hundreds of volunteers are involved. It introduces another tier of responsibility and one that provides a more personal point of contact for a larger group of volunteers than is otherwise possible. These volunteer team leaders can, for example, also organize rotas and help with induction and training. They work closely with the VSM, reporting regularly, and are a vital link to the department in which their team works. Different hospices have different formulae that work for them. One working example is St. Columba's Hospice in Edinburgh[8]. One such model is shown in Figure 3.1.

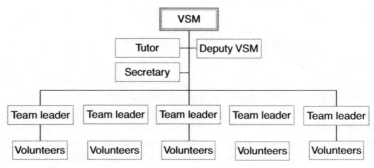

Fig. 3.1 The management structure of a volunteer service.

Other staff team members should know the appropriate lines of responsibility and communication for volunteers and be encouraged to respect the volunteer role. It may also be useful to issue a set of guidelines to help them understand how to best work alongside their volunteer colleagues. When new staff join the organization, it should be part of their induction programme to spend time with the VSM to help smooth the pathway towards working with volunteers.

Some simple features to encourage integration and a positive supportive atmosphere throughout the organization could be encouraged such as the sharing of staff rooms, social events, or a hospice internal newsletter to include both staff and volunteers.

Organizing the volunteer office

Good administrative support is essential to a successful voluntary service. Recruiting volunteers, keeping in touch with them, and valuing their involvement with the organization, can all be enhanced with efficient systems and record keeping. Providing skilled or trained volunteers in the right place at the right time is easier when accurate and up-to-date information is to hand. Planning for future projects or writing reports becomes more effective with the availability of statistics and data. Office accommodation is often in short supply, unless in purpose-built units; but as a minimum, there should be sufficient space available to house the VSM and whatever staffing is agreed with access to at least one private room for interviewing volunteers.

Administrative support should be considered under the following headings:

1 Secretarial support, systems, and paperwork

2 Record keeping

3 Data collection

Secretarial support, systems, and paperwork

Whatever resources are available, it is important to take time to plan carefully what the needs of the department are, how best to deploy the office resources available, and to design and develop efficient systems and procedures to help achieve high standards. Whether paperwork or computer systems are used, it is vitally important that procedures are simple, clear, logical, and consistent.

A high priority should be the appointment of a specific member of staff to oversee and coordinate the administrative systems in the volunteer office. This person should demonstrate a responsive and consistent approach, high levels of computer skills, and provide supervision for any extra volunteer administrative help. These will allow the VSM freedom from the minutiae of departmental organization. It is vital that the VSM does not attempt personally to undertake the administrative role. Much of the administrative support can, if there is no other alternative, be carried out by volunteers.

The VSM should not be afraid to delegate to volunteers such tasks as rota preparation, driving schedules, correspondence and liaison with other volunteers, meetings and training organization, and administration of recruitment and selection. Since a number of different volunteers may have to be involved at any one time, it is doubly important that the procedures in place are very clearly laid out and explained, that each volunteer knows exactly what is expected of them, and who to report to in the case of any difficulties. Some volunteers will be happy to play a leading role, taking on more responsibility, perhaps in a supervisory capacity, while others will be happy to be directed to do some of the more straightforward tasks[8].

If volunteers are to be involved in undertaking the many administration tasks, it is then important to ensure that sufficient resources are available to accommodate a number of different people using equipment, such as telephones, computers, desks, chairs, etc.—perhaps at the same time as each other! Involving volunteers is not necessarily a cheap option!

Investing in computer equipment and relevant software packages is a basic require-ment. Currently in the United Kingdom, new software programs are available, whilst some hospices, with the help of a resident expert (voluntary or staff), have developed their own packages. Whatever determines the decision taken, it is important that the organization has ready access to expertise to troubleshoot and develop the program to meet new requirements as these occur. Careful planning is key before committing to what might seem an expensive system. However, the benefits recouped in time and from the capability of a well-designed database, for example, will soon repay the outlay.

Record keeping

As in human resources departments, a personal file should be kept for each individual volunteer. This should include such documents as the completed applica-tion form, references, interview documentation, and any subsequent paperwork in relation to the organization. Storage of these and access to them should be in line with legislative and organizational guidelines (e.g. data protection).

Additional record-keeping systems will be developed according to the needs of the department. For example, the storing of detailed information on individual skills on offer from each volunteer, such as musical instruments played or languages spoken, may facilitate a speedy matching up of a request for help from the organization. Keeping records of attendance and starting dates provides readily available data when looking at long service or special awards. Tracking attendance and absence can flag potential problems for a volunteer. Acknowledging birthdays or an illness is a way of valuing volunteers. Recording training sessions attended and roles undertaken makes it easy to produce volunteer profiles.

Data collection

Report writing and forward planning are two elements the role of a manager. Efficient data collection from volunteer records can provide such information as age distribu-tion of volunteers, methods of recruitment, gender split, travelling costs, hours worked, training provided, etc. A well-designed data collection process can provide a large proportion of the fundamental information and statistics required.

The outreach factor

For a long time, the focus of the work of the VSM was with the volunteers inside the hospice building. With the increasing emphasis on community fund-raising trading arms of many hospices, the involvement of volunteers has spread enormously. This has added to the pressure on the volunteer office as it is often expected that the VSM will also take responsibility for these areas, in many cases without extra resources. The introduction of these 'different' volunteers also leads to other interesting questions such as how to make them feel part of the organization, how much training to offer, whether they should be treated in the same way as the hospice-based volunteers, etc. These questions amongst others should be discussed and agreed well in advance of developments. There is no rule that states that all volunteers have to come under the same remit of the volunteer office, although it is important that there is consistency in the organization's approach to volunteers.

Working to hospice standards

Offering the highest possible quality of care to patients, carers, and families is the philosophy underpinning the work of all palliative care units. The contribution made by the volunteers and the voluntary service should aim to enhance this quality of care wherever possible. To achieve this, the volunteers must be willing to actively contribute to and support these standards of practice. This necessitates working to agreed guidelines and procedures within all departments. Establishing these with the departments concerned is the role of the VSM. Promoting the idea of working to standards should be apparent in all the volunteer documentation and communication with volunteers. A good example of this is the policy for 'confidentiality', which incorporates staff and volunteers alike.

Monitoring and evaluating the service

The organization may already have a system of audit in place but, if not, this should not prevent the volunteer department from regularly reviewing its practice and effectiveness and looking at whether this can be improved. As long as aims, principal functions, policies, and procedures are in place, standards can be set 3. Measuring what actually happens against the standards will produce information on how well targets are being met.

Continually reviewing in this way uncovers problems at an early stage, recognizes successes, promotes an open attitude to change and improvement, and can encourage participation and involvement in development from across the organization. Chapter 4 deals with quality standards in some depth and provides helpful guidance on this topic.

Conclusion

The role of the VSM is thus a complex one encompassing many diverse responsibilities and requiring someone with a wide range of skills. The most important of these are a sound knowledge base on all aspects of volunteering, the ability to communicate effectively, to inspire and motivate, followed very closely by good organizational skills. A capable and respected VSM can enable the organization to reap the benefit from a potential wealth of talent and time available in the community. A well-motivated and loyal volunteer workforce is a powerful link with that same community. Volunteers can be excellent ambassadors, educating the public about the work of the hospice and attracting new volunteers to support the hospice. The VSM is the vital link in that process.

References

1 Davis Smith, J. (1996). Should volunteers be managed? In *Voluntary Agencies, Challenges of Organization and Management* (ed. David Billis and Margaret Harris), Ch. 12. London, Macmillan.
2 'InVoLve'. *Quality Programme for Voluntary Services Departments in Palliative Care*. London, Help the Hospices.
3 Institute for Volunteering Research (IVR). (1997). *National Survey of Volunteering in the UK*. IVR, obtainable from 'AVSM', c/o Help the Hospices, 34–44 Britannia St, London, WC1X 9JG.
4 Addington-Hall, J. and Karlson, S. (2001). *Summary of a National Survey of Health Professionals and Volunteers Working in Voluntary Hospices*. London, Help the Hospices.
5 Field, D. and Johnson, I. (1993). Satisfaction and Change: A Survey of Volunteers in a Hospice Organisation. Occasional Paper No. 8, April. Trent Palliative Care Centre (UK).
6 Scheier, I. H. (1993). In *Building Staff/Volunteer Relations*, Philadelphia, USA: Energize Books.
7 Hamilton, G. (1997). Volunteering: Team leadership. *Hospice Bulletin*, April, p. 1. London, The Hospice Information Service, St. Christopher's Hospice.
8 Plant, H. (1999). Working with volunteers—Team leaders. *Hospice Bulletin*, April, p. 7. London, The Hospice Information Service, St. Christopher's Hospice.

Recommended reading

Whitewood, B. (1999). The role of the volunteer in British palliative care. *European Journal of Palliative Care*, **6**(2).

Chapter 4

Considering quality and measuring impact

Steven Howlett

Introduction

This book covers a number of themes, but each is linked by presenting some aspect of good practice for managing volunteers, and particularly good practice within hospices. Good practice, one would hope, is a step towards helping ensure that volunteers have a good experience within the hospice; it is about helping secure quality of volunteer management. What we need to consider is how we define, measure, and maintain that quality. Perhaps we should begin by defining what we mean by a good experience. Here we are talking about how a volunteer experiences working with a hospice and striving to ensure that the time volunteers spend at a hospice is effective. Volunteers should feel fulfilled in terms of the motivations that inspired them to volunteer in the first place and to do this we want volunteers to feel well-supported and managed. In turn, introducing ideas of quality assurance would mean that there are agreed standards to ensure, as far as possible, that this happens.

The tools, techniques, and the passing on of wisdom and experience that fill the chapters of this book are concerned with making this happen. The point of this should be obvious—a volunteer who is satisfied in his/her work and who feels fulfilled and supported will be happier and more likely to stay with the organization, at least in theory. There are many reasons why volunteers choose to leave organizations. Some of these will be personal—volunteers leave because of changes in their life circumstances, they move away from the area, find paid work or to pursue further or higher education, and so on. Any of these may cause a volunteer to stop volunteering. On the face of it there is little a Voluntary Services Manager (VSM) could do to stop withdrawal. VSMs can, however, ameliorate factors that may cause withdrawal when those factors are linked to how volunteering is organized. In fact, some interventions could even help when volunteers look likely to withdraw because of changes in life circumstances—helping to make volunteering opportunities more flexible to suit people who work, and so on.

We also need to consider quality over and above volunteer satisfaction. We need to think about how volunteering enhances the work of the hospice and how this is done by maintaining certain standards in terms of the work and caring which volunteers do as well as in terms of how volunteers are managed. The issues are connected, and a well-supported and satisfied volunteer ought, *ceteris paribus,* to enhance hospice work and to be trained to a level that provides a good addition to the work of the hospice.

There is a key role here for the VSM in terms of being the focal point to manage volunteers and enhance quality. This book is focussed mainly on the work of VSMs and this chapter asks some key questions around the issues of quality and impact. How do we benchmark and ensure quality? Where should quality standards be located—should it be defined at the level of the VSM or should standards be defined in terms of organizational structures and systems? Connected to this is how do we measure what is working. We will also be considering in this chapter how we measure the impact of volunteering. The two issues sit together here because we want to think about how volunteers experience their volunteering; we may expect that volunteers will have a quality experience if we have the correct quality standards in place, but how do we know? We will therefore look first at quality standards and focus on the Investing in Volunteers (IiV) award. We will then consider one way of measuring the impact of volunteering by looking at the Impact Assessment Toolkit developed by the Institute for Volunteering Research. This 'do-it-yourself' research tool enables an organization to measure and demonstrate the impact of volunteering, but at the same time gives valuable feedback on the processes of volunteering and volunteer management within an organization.

Why consider quality?

The answer to this question has been alluded to in the introduction and may seem patently obvious: of course we want to strive for quality, but what do we mean, how do we define it, and what benefits does it confer? In this chapter we are concerned in particular with volunteers and volunteer management, and quality in this context will mean achieving some sort of standard of volunteer involvement through having some indicators or measures that are clear and explicit enough for organizations to be able to compare performance against and to work towards implementing.

Inevitably, it is more complicated than this because achieving some sort of quality standard does not necessarily guarantee a successful volunteer programme. There is research that shows that quality of volunteer management does *not* cause people to quit volunteering as much as people might think and that it is more likely to be the personal reasons mentioned earlier—moving away, getting other paid work, and so on—that cause people to leave[1].

Nevertheless, there is a body of work that does suggest that quality is something VSMs ignore at their peril, even if it does not draw clear cut cause and effect lines between quality of experience and retention. The first piece of evidence to note is the often-quoted statistic that in 1997[2], 73 per cent of volunteers said that they thought their volunteering could be better organized; volunteers it seems want their work to be managed in some form. This is underscored by the work of Kathy Gaskin (mentioned in Chapter 2), which also suggests that volunteers, while eschewing over formalization, expect to be managed in a balanced way that combines a recognized need for proper organizational policy and process, with a sensitivity to the fact that volunteers are not paid and so should not always be managed as paid workers are[3]. Combined with this is research that argues volunteer management needs to draw on a range of functions including person management, task management, acting as the trainer, being a skilled administrator, and so on in order to fulfil the role effectively[4].

All this is underlined by more common sense thinking—volunteers will work best when their roles and experience are looked after by a competent supervisor of some sort. This is neatly summed up by one report, which observed that although volunteers might find intrinsic benefits from being volunteers, organizations also have a role to play in getting management right:

> 'Virtue might be its "own reward" but intelligent and progressive management practices would not hurt either'[5]

On the one hand, therefore, we have an argument that managing volunteers cannot guarantee that volunteers will enjoy the experience and stay with an organization longer, but on the other hand is evidence that it helps, and it helps when volunteers are managed in an appropriate style. The task is to somehow convey how to manage in this appropriate style. Best practices at this can then be set as standards, which convey quality management.

While a key motivation for establishing consistent good practice through putting systems in place is aimed at the volunteer experience, the process of thinking about quality can also perform a number of other functions; it can:

◆ Focus attention on what the organization is doing. In volunteer management, this can usefully question those aspects which an organization does because 'we have always done it this way'; going through a quality assessment helps question assumptions and compares procedure against benchmarks of good practice.

◆ Help build teams by focussing organizations on areas and functions of the volunteer programme and requires collective thinking to ensure policies are present and up to standard.

◆ Ensure that stakeholders also see that the organization and its functions are of a quality standard.

◆ Help the planning process and acts as a benchmark for future development.

Defining quality standards

The adoption of quality standards has a history that has been shown to have begun in manufacturing and gradually permeated through the public and voluntary sectors. Within the voluntary and community sector, this has been linked to ideas of accountability, user involvement, and performance of organizations[6]. There is now a proliferation of quality standards and marks an organization can access. For example, IiV concentrates on volunteer involvement and which we explore in the following paragraphs. Other standards can be broadly grouped into two: those that are general to all organizations and which include volunteering as one function among other organizational functions or those that are aimed at particular sub-sectors. The former group includes Investors in People, which looks at all staff, of which volunteers are considered to be a subset, and PQASSO, which includes managing volunteers among a range of topics (including, for example, managing money and communications). The latter group includes, for example, the Approved Provider Standard (APS), which is a national benchmark for organizations providing one-to-one volunteer mentoring or befriending, and Reach, which is designed for youth action agencies.

We will look in a bit more detail at IiV in the following paragraphs, but first we will consider some thinking that organizations will need to do before choosing a quality mark and how to engage with the standard:

- The first step seems obvious; decide which standard the organization wants to go for. This chapter assumes that the VSM will concentrate on volunteering, but a hospice might want to consider Investors in People as a quality measure for the whole organization.

- The setting up of a working group encourages commitment to the standard and increases the effectiveness of the process. This may include the VSM, those who work with volunteers, others within the hospice who have a personnel function, and also representatives of volunteers.

- The process needs to be completed in an environment of openness and which encourages problem identification and solving. Research has suggested that implementation problems tend to be operational rather than ideological[7].

- Organizations will also want to consider cost, whether advisors are available to help with the process, or whether organizations are more self-assessed. It is suggested that it is sensible to talk to other groups using quality systems.

Investing in Volunteers (IiV)

We will now look at IiV on the assumption that VSMs will, in particular, be looking at how to assess quality systems within their own function area. This section will not look in detail at the award; it is not appropriate here to do that because not all readers will have access to the award, which is run by Volunteering England. Details of the programme can be found at http://www.investinginvolunteers.org.uk. Neither is there the space to talk through the award, rather we will look at some of the general issues around the award. For this, we will draw on an evaluation of the award[8].

The origins of IiV show very clearly why quality marks are a good idea. Four volunteer centres in south London realized that although they were assiduously performing their function of matching volunteers to opportunities, they had no way, other than feedback from volunteers or visiting centre staff, to be sure that the organizations they directed volunteers to were able to give volunteers a good experience. They developed a pilot scheme with a view to it being evaluated and modified for a possible national roll-out. The evaluation showed that the award was highly thought of by organizations but that there were some reservations about the amount of work needed to complete the award. When Volunteering England stepped in to take the award national, the indicators were rationalized in order to make the process more manageable for organizations.

What IiV covers

Although we are not looking in great detail at the award, it is useful to note what it covers.

The relevance of the award is centred around concentrating on four main areas of management, namely planning for involvement; recruiting; selecting and matching, and supporting and retaining.

The standard is based around ten indicators. These are:

Indicator 1. There is an expressed commitment to the involvement of volunteers, and recognition throughout the organization that volunteering is a two-way process, which benefits volunteers and the organization.

Indicator 2. The organization commits appropriate resources to working with volunteers, such as money, management, staff time, and materials.

Indicator 3. The organization is open to involving volunteers who reflect the diversity of the local community, in accordance with the organization's stated aims, and operates procedures.

Indicator 4. The organization develops appropriate roles for volunteers in line with its aims and objectives, and which are of value to the volunteers and create an environment where they can develop.

Indicator 5. The organization is committed to ensuring that, as far as possible, volunteers are protected from physical, financial, and emotional harm arising from volunteering.

Indicator 6. The organization is committed to using fair, efficient, and consistent recruitment procedures for all potential volunteers.

Indicator 7. The organization takes a considered approach to taking up references and official checks which is consistent and equitable for all volunteers, bearing in mind the nature of the work.

Indicator 8. Clear procedures are put into action for introducing new volunteers to the organization, its work, policies, practices, and relevant personnel.

Indicator 9. Everybody in the organization is aware of the need to give volunteers recognition.

Indicator 10. The organization takes account of the varying support needs of volunteers.

Each of these indicators has 'practices attached' of which there are 55 in total. So, for example, Indicator 1 has four practices. As an example, practice 1 states:

> *The organization has a written policy on volunteer involvement, based on equal opportunities principles, which sets out the procedures for recruiting, supporting, and protecting volunteers*

When an organization enrols for the award they are assigned an assessor who, when it comes to consider whether the organization has reached the quality standard required, will look for evidence for each practice. So, to assess the practice outlined earlier, the assessor may look for policy documents such as, for example, a volunteer policy.

Working through the indicators enables an organization to examine practice and put into place systems and procedures that are missing or strengthen existing practice which does not meet the standard. It also offers a way of documenting what seems to work in practice, which the hospice might find difficult to show. Indeed demonstrating professionalism and good practice was one of the motivating decisions that encouraged organizations to take part alongside providing them with a clear structure to which they could work[8].

Challenges and changes

The standard does prove challenging to organizations and the volume of work to develop new systems was one area that organizations drew researchers attention to[8]. A positive aspect of this, however, may be how it is related to one of the issues noted earlier—organizations reported that working towards the standard was useful for them to bring systems to an acceptable level. The volume of work needed is therefore an expression of the importance of the work; any organization needing to put in a lot of work will probably reflect that it showed that their approach to management did need scrutiny and tightening up.

Another challenge noted was the cost of the process[8]. There is no denying that putting an organization through quality standards does cost money, but this underscores the importance of realizing that volunteering is not a free resource; it is cost-effective, but not cost free. While this is a point VSMs will be aware of, it is a message senior management teams and boards of trustees sometimes need reminding of. Factoring in cost may be one of the criteria which helps hospices decide what quality system they want to pursue.

The evidence of the research was that the organizations interviewed made several changes to their management practices. Alongside general modifications of policies was the introduction of regular reviews, altered and new recruitment methods, increased training, and improvement in information-giving and greater attention to issues of diversity and risk assessment.

Interestingly, volunteers interviewed were generally supportive of the process but did not see the relevance to them[8]. This may not be a negative view, however. It is certainly the experience of the author in researching volunteering that while volunteers want to be well organized, they do not necessarily want to see themselves as managed—good management is often that which facilitates happy and productive volunteers while not being highly visible.

Locating expertise

So far we have looked at alternative quality frameworks. Each of these assesses quality in terms of organizational procedure. The implication seems to be that having systems in place would mean that anybody could assume the role of VSM and run the volunteers by operating the system. And yet, something tells us that the job of the VSM is different, it implies a broad range of skills as we noted earlier, from the organization of administration to the diplomacy of a skilled people manager. So instead of locating quality and know-how within the systems of an organization, could we look at instilling quality checks within each VSM?

On the one hand, volunteer management is not a profession in the same sense doctors and lawyers are, but it is to the extent that it involves some degree of specialist knowledge and proficiency. But how do we measure that knowledge? How does anyone new to the role of the VSM know what level of tasks is expected of them? One answer comes through the National Occupational Standards for Volunteers Management, which was published in 2004 by the Voluntary Sector National Training Organization and updated in 2008. It was the result of consultation with a great many individuals across the United Kingdom who manage and coordinate volunteers. As a result, the standard can be used to review practice and plan professional development. The standards can be used:

- As a checklist for measuring their own performance.
- To identify professional development needs within their role and to help career progression.
- To accumulate evidence that may lead to a nationally-recognized qualification (but only where an N/SVQ exists and where agreed to by the Body)[9].

It isn't either/or

In fact the extensive standards compliment IiV so that VSMs can measure their own development alongside that of the organization. It is important that VSMs see their own development as crucial to the well-being of volunteers. Chapter 2 noted the trend in volunteering to greater formalization and argued that while in some circumstances this was needed, there are times when formalization threatens the simplicity of volunteering—of one person giving of their time to help a cause. The imposition of standards can seem to be exacerbating this, but a VSM confident in their knowledge and skills becomes a key element in ensuring volunteer programmes are successful. For example, good practice suggests that volunteers are regularly supervised—but a good VSM knows that a policy of regular supervision can range from a formal meeting for volunteers who are engaged in highly skilled or possibly emotionally draining roles, to having a cup of tea and a chat to see how things are going with the volunteers who run the shop.

Standards are a clear way of benchmarking practice, but they are not the only form of support a VSM gets. Support can and should come from within the hospice, but many VSMs will also want to enhance their knowledge and share experience with peers, this is where new developments like the Association of Volunteer Managers have a role to play—as an organization that supports volunteer managers but also acts as a voice for the developing profession[10].

Volunteer impact—measuring our volunteer programmes

Establishing quality measures should help improve the management of volunteers. But even so, how can we be sure that our volunteer programme is working well and achieving its desired effects? One way is to evaluate our volunteer programme. This chapter looks at how we might do this by addressing another important indicator of volunteer success—impact. We will use the remainder of this chapter to explore a tool to look at the impact of volunteering, but one which also provides valuable management data.

Volunteer-involving organizations are not only frequently asked to show how they deliver on quality, but also to demonstrate what difference they make. This can be a tough ask as many organizations are not familiar with techniques to think about measuring impact. Prompted by this, the Institute for Volunteering Research developed the 'Volunteering Impact Assessment Toolkit' (VIAT), a 'D-I-Y' assessment of the impact of volunteering across a range of stakeholders. The toolkit starts by recognizing that the need to show impact comes from several directions including:

- Demand from funders who increasingly want to know what difference their funding makes.
- Demand from organizations that want to know what works and what could work better.
- Demand from volunteers recognizing that 'no one wants to give their time to something that has no impact'.
- A general need for ways to demonstrate actions that could show accountability.
- Providing management data to facilitate organizational learning.

Moreover, measuring, impacts can have beneficial affects within and outside the organization:

Internal:

- A greater understanding of what works and a sound basis for planning and strategy.
- Feedback to staff on the impacts and benefits of their work.
- Re-balancing priorities and the allocation of resources among different area of work.

External:

- Feedback from your users and stakeholders that can strengthen relationships and enhance your performance.
- Accountability to funders on the outcomes and impacts of your work.
- Evidence to attract new funding.
- Accountability to the local volunteering sector and community.
- Promotion and public relations to raise your profile and attract users.
- Information for governments and policy makers to support the case for an effective, well-resourced volunteering infrastructure.

How the toolkit works

The toolkit offers a range of research tools, for example, survey questionnaires, interview discussion guides, and focus group discussion guides and activities to help organizations assess the impact of volunteering. It considers a range of stakeholders noting that volunteering will have an impact in a number of areas:

- On volunteers
- On organizations
- On service users
- On the wider community

Volunteers

Volunteers mostly tell us they volunteer because they enjoy it—but how can we describe their enjoyment and dig deeper to see what difference volunteering makes? We may look for increased feelings of well-being or through access to wider networks of social contacts. We might measure the skills volunteers learn—are they hard skills gained from a particular task, or softer transferable skills like communication, organization, and leadership? Are there benefits to be had in the paid-labour market? Has volunteering helped volunteers get paid work or helped them progress in their paid work maybe through promotion? There are a whole range of ways in which volunteers can benefit.

Volunteer-involving organizations and their staff

Similarly, the organizations that involve volunteers can be impacted upon; for example, volunteers might bring additional skills, viewpoints, or add to the diversity of an organization. Volunteers can enable the organization to deliver services over and above what they could deliver with paid staff alone. The toolkit looks to measure these and has a template to work out the notional 'value' of volunteering. Readers may be familiar with the Volunteer Investment and Value Audit (VIVA)[11], which expresses the 'return' organizations get for every pound they invest and this forms the basis of the template within the VIAT. This can be a powerful way of expressing what volunteering means to the hospice. A study for Help The Hospices, for example, using the VIVA on a selection of hospices, estimated that that the value of volunteering across all independent charitable hospices was some £122 million[12].

Service users

Service users also benefit from volunteer input. In the case of hospices, this will be the patient and their family.

With some thought, we can start to identify all sorts of impacts on patients and families. We might consider, for example, how volunteers increase the well-being and self esteem; reduce stress and anxiety in patients and their families.

Communities

We can also think in terms of benefits and impacts on the wider community. Researching these impacts takes time and resources, so this may be one area that hospices do not want to devote time to discovering, but the toolkit helps organizations do this should they want to. It might not be just a physical community we want to research. For example, the presence of a hospice with extensive volunteer input might be something that local people feel demonstrates how the communities cares for itself, but it might also be that we want to show how volunteering adds to a community of health-care professionals. Examples from outside of the United Kingdom show how projects organized to give palliative care can have a huge impact on communities and indeed be community led.

Across each of these stakeholder groups there are five different areas over which benefits can be seen. The VIAT calls them 'capitals' to imply that volunteering banks a store of something as a result of participation. These areas are:

◆ Economic capital
◆ Physical capital
◆ Human capital

◆ Social capital
◆ Cultural capital

Economic capital

This measures how volunteering adds economically across the stakeholder groups. So, for example, volunteers can benefit economically because they may access training as part of their volunteering and that has a value attached to it, or they become employed after volunteering. These measures (and others) begin to build up a picture of how a project adds to economic well-being.

In terms of the organization, the VIVA measure would show just how much an organization benefits from volunteer input by supposing the roles taken by volunteers had to be paid for and calculating how much an organization would have to pay to get the work done.

Physical capital

This is a measure of the physical things volunteers are involved with—suppose, for example, volunteers helped in a hospice garden, what did they plant, build, and repair? But it could relate to other services—how many car trips did volunteers do to take patients to appointments and home again, or how many hair-dressing sessions were held.

Human capital

Here we would want look at the skills volunteers acquired, or that they passed on to others in the community. What were those skills and how did people benefit from them, what did they use them for? In short how does the volunteer, service user, organization, and community benefit from the increase in skills.

Social capital

In contrast to physical capital, which looks at inanimate objects and human capital, which tries to tease out the skills individuals acquire and use, social capital is more about relationships between people and communities. Social capital has been rather fashionable within academic and policy circles for some time and tries to look at how volunteering increases trust between people and influences what are referred to as norms of behaviour, which are said to develop out of relationships that form as people work together.

Cultural capital

Cultural capital refers to shared senses of cultural meaning such as religious identity or language. It is the measure organizations are perhaps least likely to focus on, but can demonstrate how volunteering brings people together and strengthens particular features of a group or community, or indeed links different groups through sharing experience.

Bringing the elements together

The VIAT is very practical in that it provides tools for each stakeholder across each measure—so, for example, sample questions and measures are available for looking at the economic, physical, social, human, and cultural impact for volunteers, for organizations, services users, and the wider community. In practice, organizations might focus on only one element and measure that with a view to repeating the process after a period of time to assess progress, or focus on one element one year and another area the next.

In terms of where we started this chapter—looking at quality, using the VIAT can give a strong idea of how the volunteer programme is working and allow improvements to be developed.

Ros Scott, editor of this volume, used the VIAT to assess volunteering at the Children's Hospice Association Scotland (CHAS). Ros was able to look at all areas of the CHAS volunteer programme. This was a big task, but made manageable by involving volunteers as researchers to collect data. Volunteers were trained to undertake assessment on staff, volunteers, and service users.

The results showed that[13]:

Volunteers: positive experience. Eighty-four per cent said they had built friendships and networks through volunteering, but 18 per cent felt their skills weren't being utilized.

Staff: valued the role of volunteers. Eighty-three per cent felt volunteers helped create open and diverse culture, but 18 per cent felt they were over reliant on volunteers, and some did not recognize board members as volunteers.

Families: significant impact of volunteers on families. Seventy-three per cent said volunteers led to new friendships and social networks, but some were concerned about how volunteers were vetted and whether they should be undertaking care roles.

From this the hospice was able to draw up a number of recommendations, which helped build a new strategy:

◆ Review how volunteer skills are utilized to full effect.

◆ Raise awareness within the organization of the role and volunteer status of the board.

◆ Explore the possibility of extending volunteer roles to home-care support.

In addition, the research has been presented within CHAS and externally and specific areas of practice were developed based on the findings, for example:

◆ A leaflet for families about volunteers, their role, and how they are recruited.

◆ A review of volunteer role descriptions.

Conclusions

This chapter has looked at two areas—quality and impact. Quality measures allow VSMs to benchmark good practice. Different models exist and organizations need to choose carefully which is best for them. But quality cannot stand still, and when organizations achieve quality measures, VSMs still need to ensure that they work! By looking at measuring impact we are able to follow through what difference volunteer programmes make—a useful exercise for a number of reasons. Exploring the Volunteer Impact Assessment Toolkit (VIAT) we were able to see that as well as providing useful data for funders, volunteers, and service users, the process also gives us information that can help inform and improve our management practices.

References

1　Machin, J. and Ellis Paine, A. (2008). *Management Matters: A National Survey of Volunteer Management Capacity*. London, Institute for Volunteering Research.

2　Davis Smith, J. (1998). *The 1997 National Survey of Volunteering*. London, National Centre for Volunteering.

3　Gaskin, K. (2003). *A Choice Blend: What Volunteers Want from Organisation and Management*. London, Institute for Volunteering Research.

4　Gay, P. (2000). *Delivering the Goods: A Report of the Work of Volunteer Managers*. London, Institute for Volunteering Research.

5　Penner, L. (2002). 'Dispositional and Organizational Influences on Sustained Volunteerism: An Interactionist Perspective'. *Journal of Social Issues* **58**(3), 447–467, page 464 quoted in Rochester, C., Ellis Paine, A., and Howlett, S. (2009). *Volunteering in the 21st Century*, Basingstoke, Palgrave, which discusses retention and management issues in more depth with reference to research material.

6　Cains, B. and Hutchinson, R. (2006). *The Impact of Investing in Volunteers*. Birmingham, Aston Business School.

7　Cairns, B., Hutchinson, R., and Schofiled, J. (2004). *The Adoption and Use of Quality Systems in the Voluntary Sector*. Exective summary available for download at http://www.ivar.org.uk/documents/Quality_ExecSummary.pdf

8　Cairns, B. and Hutchinson, R. (2006). *op cit*

9　http://www.ukworkforcehub.org.uk/component/content/article/266

10　http://www.volunteermanagers.org.uk/ it should be noted that AVM is an England wide organisation.

11　Gaskin, K. (1999a). *VIVA in Europe: A Comparative Study of the Volunteer Investment and Value Audit*, London, Institute for Volunteering Research.

12　http://www.helpthehospices.org.uk/our-services/hospice-volunteers-and-volunteering/publications/

13　Scott, R. (2006). 'Volunteers in a Children's Hospice'. *Voluntary Action* **8**(2), 55–63.

Chapter 5

The selection of volunteers

Sally-Ann Spencer-Gray

Why do we need a process of selection?

Palliative care and specialist palliative care provision involves working at the 'sharp end' of health care, with people made vulnerable through illness and an unrelenting prognosis. This care may be provided through a charity, private or government-funded health-care provisions, all of which may involve volunteers to enhance/complement their service. Regardless of funding, the patients, their carers, and families have expectations of palliative care services to provide quality care and support, safely and competently adhering to national and international standards.

In the selection of volunteers we are:

* Exercising a legal and moral obligation, a duty of care.

* Choosing the best and most appropriate people for our organization.

* Not just choosing the right people but choosing the right people at the right time for both the organization and the individual.

* Identifying potential, looking for those who have the capacity for development and growth—who will blossom in and enhance the palliative care environment.

* Protecting to the best of our ability those people in the organization's care—patients, carers, paid staff, and volunteers—from physical, emotional, and spiritual harm.

Poor selection of volunteers can lead to disruption, conflict, and harm to individuals and the organization.

According to Smith[1] an organization can adopt one of three selection approaches but these can often overlap:

1 *Non-rejection*—nobody is rejected because there is always some job suitable.

2 *Recruitment*—recruited and selected for a specific task only—similar to paid employment techniques.

3 *Matching*—looking at what the volunteer is presenting and finding a job to match.

The selection of volunteers can fit into three main groups:

1 Recruited (active recruitment by the hospice):

* Blanket recruitment (a general appeal for volunteers)

* Recruitment for a specific area of work, for example, day care or for a specific task (e.g. as a driver)

2 Unsolicited applications: Individuals or groups independent of recruitment drives approach the organization with a wish to volunteer, with or without a specific task in mind.

3 Work experience/student training placements/government schemes: These can be at the individual's request or a condition of qualifying either for training/employment or for government benefits, e.g. unemployment benefits.

The selection process

Selection is a dynamic process—it has specific criteria that must be met along the way but it also enables some flexibility to accommodate individual circumstances and professional judgement. The selection process consists of the following components, the order of which will vary with organizational policy and personal preference:

- Application
- References
- Interview
- Induction
- Probationary period

Throughout the process of selection the voluntary services manager (VSM) uses a combination of:

- Interpersonal and communication skills
- Experience
- Professional judgement
- Discretion
- Intuition
- Gut feeling

Judgement is needed to determine the weight of each factor as it is presented. Written, verbal, and non-verbal communications are examined in order to make a value judgement whilst ensuring that he/she and other members of staff are not being manipulated.

Box 5.1 Some of the skills needed by a VSM when selecting volunteers

- Informal and formal interview technique and skills—interpretation of verbal and non-verbal messages
- Using open and closed questions
- Basic counselling/communication skills—listening, empathy, paraphrasing or rephrasing, summarizing, giving feedback
- Breaking bad news—handling and understanding rejection

There are five stages in the selection process, which are clearly illustrated in Fig. 5.1 and Fig. 5.2. The crucially important difference between the two is when confidential reports or references are called for and used. Some interviewers prefer to have seen them and have them in front of them when they see the applicant. Others only call for them after the interview. There are points in favour of each.

The selection process is an opportunity for both the organization and the volunteer to decide if they are suited to each other and that the selection process permits rejection as well as selection. Rejection, for whatever reason, may take place at various

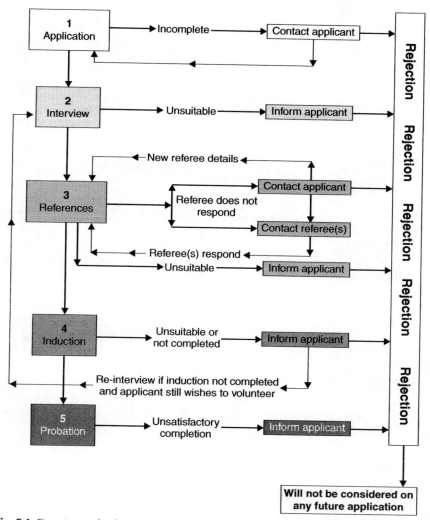

Fig. 5.1 Five-stage selection criteria. Interview before references requested. (From S.A. Spencer Gray, 2001.)

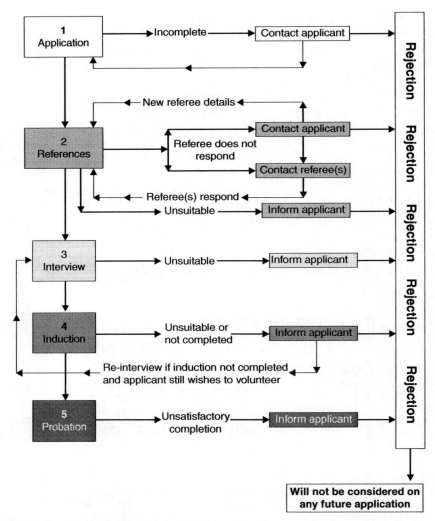

Fig. 5.2 Five-stage selection criteria. Interview with references already provided. (From S.A. Spencer Gray, 2001.)

stages of the process, as illustrated in Fig. 5.1 and Fig. 5.2 and discussed in the following paragraphs.

The basis for selection

The VSM and management colleagues must decide on what will they judge the suitability of an applicant. Will it be primarily on the:

◆ Application form?
◆ Past history?

◆ References?

◆ Interview—information ascertained and gut feeling?

Application

Application will involve the completion of an application form either written or submitted electronically by secure means to ensure confidentiality. A designated person must be made responsible for applications coming in, for acknowledging them, and for calling for references, to ensure confidentiality and best practice.

The application form differs from the forms used to employ paid staff but should observe a similar equal opportunity, non-discriminatory, confidential approach. In general, the emphasis will be on life experience, skills, and motivation rather than on qualifications. However, when recruiting for a specific task or an application to work in a 'qualified' capacity (e.g. complementary therapies), then specific qualifications will be required that meet with an agreed/approved competency pathway (i.e. a minimum requirement of professional bodies and/or the organization).

An equal opportunities statement must be included on the form—non-discriminatory with regard to gender, sexual orientation, creed, colour, religion, level of ability or disability. Carefully thought-out 'open' questions should be used where possible, with strategically placed closed questions to prevent ambiguity in crucial areas (e.g. criminal convictions). The questions should be kept to a minimum.

Box 5.2 Open and closed questions

An example of an open question:
'Why you would like to help at the hospice'

Will elicit a descriptive answer.

An example of a closed question:
'Do you have a criminal conviction?'

Will elicit a yes or no answer.

What is the minimum information you need to get from this form?

◆ Name

◆ Address

◆ Health status

◆ Criminal convictions

◆ Motivation

◆ What they would like to do to help

◆ Names and addresses of two referees

What is the minimum information you will give with this form?

◆ Organizational details—name, address etc., registered charity number.

◆ Name and job title of contact person.

- Confidentiality explanation—regarding details given by the applicant and regarding the nature of hospice work. (Some organizations include a confidentiality statement to be signed and returned with the application form. It would be better practice to sign this statement at a later stage after the meaning and implications of confidentiality have been carefully discussed with the volunteer.)
- Mention should be made of the particular stresses that can be encountered in hospice work and palliative care—alluding to recent bereavement, etc. (This can be done either on the application form or in an accompanying leaflet that gives details of volunteer opportunities available, etc.)
- A brief explanation as to who to give as a referee.
- The need for honesty and openness (e.g. declaring criminal convictions).

The language used in these forms will be less formal than normally used in application forms, with explanations accompanying terminology to ensure they are easy to understand, feel non-threatening, and encourage openness and honesty. It may be worth having the application form and explanatory notes checked for 'Plain English'[2] to ensure that the language used has been kept simple and straightforward.

Those people with poor literacy skills or sensory impairment may need assistance with the completion of their application forms. This can be facilitated by:

- Applicant being accompanied/assisted by a witness/advocate.
- Audio or videotape recordings of application interviews.

In the case of an incomplete or unsatisfactory completion of the application form, contact the applicant—by letter or telephone, providing a contact name and number: either requesting more information or the name of another referee or informing the applicant they have been unsuccessful this time.

Such phone calls can be difficult. Document them in the applicant's notes or in their computer entry. If it is considered a difficult call (having decided that it really is necessary in the first place), then it may be recorded with the applicant having been informed, or conducted in the hearing of others, again with the applicant having been informed. Permission or consent for witnesses or recording from the applicant is not necessary but they must be informed of any action you are taking.

> **Key issue:** This is the first point in the selection process when an applicant may be rejected.

References/confidential reports

Usually two references or 'confidential reports' will be required. The purpose of these references and the assurance of confidentiality must be made clear to the applicant.

If possible, one of these referees should be their current or last employer but otherwise they can be friends or colleagues but they cannot be relatives. Some organizations may call for a doctor's reference and some may tailor their references to the job involved.

It is the responsibility of the prospective employer, not the applicant, to call for these reports from the people named by the applicant.

> **Key issue:** Do you request references before or after interview? What are the 'pros' and 'cons'?

Calling for references

- Use a standard letter requesting references and enclose a standard form.
- Enclose a 'prepaid' addressed envelope (makes it easier to return).
- Listen to verbal/telephone references (they may prefer to speak to someone rather than fill in forms).
- Act on verbal leads where appropriate.
- Do not accept letters of recommendation presented by the applicant without further verification.

> **Key issue:** Do you inform the applicant that rejection was because of a confidential report? How much information do you give about it? Will it embarrass the person providing the report? Should you inform the referee of the rejection?

Interview

The interview suggested here takes place *before* induction but it is appreciated that this will not be every organization's policy. Other options include:

- Interview after induction; and.
- Interviews before and after induction.

The interview is often called an 'informal interview', 'a meeting', or 'a visit' to make it feel less threatening. There are two ways of identifying suitability for interview (see Figure 5.1 and Figure 5.2):

- From information provided on the application form.
- From such information plus information from references.

The approach adopted will depend on personal preference and organizational policy. In either option, the interview may have been conducted at the same time as completion of the application form if assistance with this was required. Progression to induction will still depend on receipt of suitable references. Depending on the volunteer role, consideration will also be required regarding the undertaking of criminal record (disclosure) checks in line with current legislation.

Selection by interview *before* induction can prevent waste of time and money for both the organization and the applicant. It may also prevent feelings of resentment in unsuccessful applicants who felt that going through an induction was equated with acceptance. This in turn helps to preserve the good name of the organization and demonstrates good practice.

It is worth remembering that people volunteer for a reason and that reason needs to be ascertained. Putting applicants at ease helps the VSM to discover that reason. *The interview itself should be as informal as possible.* It should:

- Put people at their ease.
- Encourage spontaneous divulging of information—often of a personal nature.
- Allow applicants to express their personality.
- Allow for expression of feelings—about themselves, others, and situations.
- Allow for expression of beliefs—religious and non-religious, values—what they hold dear and attitudes—their opinions, their way of thinking and behaving.
- Enable investigation and discussion of motivation. Why are they here, what do they want from the experience, what do they feel they can contribute?

Considerations when conducting an informal interview are:

- Preparation
- The venue
- Who will be present/conduct the interview?
- Interview structure
- Equity

These approaches are common to managing volunteers in many organizations and some of these issues are further discussed by Steve McCurley and Rick Lynch in their book[3]. It is useful to stress that the interview should be informal. The tendency for management to be formal was noted in Chapter 2 and there can be a real tension between having robust systems and appearing to be 'too bureaucratic' to volunteers. The interview process is an example of how a VSM can mitigate this by having procedures in place but presenting then in a more informal way when talking with volunteers.

Preparation

- Arrange interview times with space between interviews to allow for delays and some thinking time.
- Book and prepare the venue—availability, comfortable chairs, refreshments, etc.
- Have the volunteer's information present—application form, references—read these before the interview.
- Have a list of the jobs available with descriptions and required criteria.
- Have your questions prepared—there will be general questions and job/task specific ones—are you going to use an interview record form?
- Have information available to give to the potential volunteers about their chosen area of work, the organization, and confidentiality—should they sign a confidentiality statement at this time?

The venue

The interview may be conducted in an office, a designated interview or counselling room designed to ensure privacy; comfort; and uninterrupted 'quality time'. If the volunteer feels they are in the way, being rushed, or they are being interviewed in an open or shared office, they will not feel valued. If they are made to feel unimportant they are less likely to 'open up' and will not form a favourable opinion of the person conducting the interview or ultimately of the organization. First impressions last!

Who is going to be present/conduct the interview?

It is desirable to have two people to interview to try to minimize subjectivity, but again VSMs must also be aware of how this appears to a prospective volunteer—a panel can seem daunting. Part of the skill a VSM needs is to be able to balance the formal and informal. If you are interviewing for a specific post or role it might be advantageous to collaborate with the line manager/supervisor there as well. This will ensure that all the needs of the post are being met, the staff are happy with the allocation, and it also improves interdepartmental relationships.

The interviewer will normally be the VSM or a person designated by him/her to conduct interviews in his/her absence. The interviewer must have some interview knowledge and skills training.

Interview structure

An interview has a beginning, a middle, and an end.

The *beginning* or opening—build a rapport and put the interviewee at their ease

- ◆ Make the volunteer feel welcome, and thank him/her for showing an interest in the organization and taking the time to attend.

- ◆ Explain the purpose of the interview—to find out more about each other (organization and volunteer), to identify any suitable positions for that individual, and to come to a decision (mutual) as to the suitability of volunteering with this organization. Ensure the volunteer knows he/she is free to ask questions at any time during the interview process.

As previously stated, selection is a two-way process that belongs as much to the volunteer as to the organization. The volunteer can reject the organization. If it is considered that the applicant is unsuitable you can subtly and constructively steer the opinions and discussion so that it is the volunteer that chooses not to continue with the application.

The *middle*—information exchange and assessment/appraisal of the volunteer

- ◆ Here, detailed information about the work of the hospice is given to include confidentiality, the sensitive nature of this work, and some of the particular stress or consequences of the job (e.g. bereavement). Available jobs are discussed to include their importance to the organization and to the patients, identifying the skills, and/ or qualifications needed for each.

- ◆ Most of the interview is going to be about getting the volunteers to talk about themselves, their interests, their skills, and their motivation. Give volunteers time to discuss the available jobs. How would they approach the work? What training do they feel they need? This can give some insight into attitudes to the hospice/ work/patients involved and also shows how they perceive themselves and their needs.

◆ Looking out for different personality traits can help you identify a job match for a volunteer and can also help to assess suitability for volunteering. There are many different areas to look out for whilst interviewing. For example:

- Ease in answering questions about personal attributes and background—are they trying to hide something, are they embarrassed by a lack of qualifications?
- Ability to communicate well—do they use inappropriate language, do they have difficulty in expressing themselves?
- Level of enthusiasm and commitment. General attitudes and emotional reactions— do they show overwhelming emotion or prejudices?
- Types of questions they ask about the organization and the position on offer— does this seem a healthy interest?
- Other interests and hobbies—life should be about balance. If the individual does not seem to have any other interests in life and they want to commit most of their time to the organization it has to be questioned is this healthy for them and the organization?
- Flexibility and reliability. Maturity and stability—this is not always associated with age.
- Do they want to work as part of a team—does this have implications for team working, for supervision, and for taking instruction?
- Level of self-confidence—do they seem lacking in confidence or do they seem over-confident and 'know it all'? Any sense of a hidden agenda—can you tackle them about this?
- Patterns in previous jobs and volunteering—do they show poor attendance or unreliability? Reasons for coming to the interview—genuine wish to volunteer, because they were told to in order to claim benefits etc., just to see what the hospice was about? To gain some interview experience?
- Preferences in type of work—a volunteer can be adamant about patient contact or bereavement counselling when this is clearly unsuitable given their references, skills and personal history—this shows poor self-awareness or may indicate a hidden agenda? A volunteer wanting no patient contact at all (e.g. wanting to work in one of the charity shops) perhaps can be better understood.

Although each interview will be tailored to the individual, the same areas of discussion and information will be included each time. The use of an interview form will help maintain quality, consistency, and equity.

The end At the end of the interview what are you offering?—a role? induction? training (e.g. as a bereavement support volunteer)? Give clear details of the next stage of the process with time scales and expectations.

In the case of training as a bereavement support volunteer, home care visitor, etc., it must be made clear that a further selection interview is necessary after successful completion of their training. The training will not automatically guarantee that individual a position in that area of work.

Equity

To 'treat everybody the same' does not provide equity. Equity in this instance means that regardless of socioeconomic status, race, gender, sexual orientation, ethnicity, culture, and/or disability, an individual will have equal opportunity to access information about and be able to apply to be and have equal chance of selection as a volunteer. Equity actions are deliberate efforts to ensure that services and information are flexible in form and function to ensure equal access to all—they eliminate bias, stereotyping, and discrimination. Access for all will permeate all aspects of the hospice and palliative care provision and will adhere to statutory obligations (Acts of Law) and to your organization's equal opportunities policy and code of conduct. Selection criteria for all posts must be clearly defined and reflected in the information sent to applicants, which must also include details of the organization's commitment to equality of opportunity.

The interview is the second point in the selection process when an applicant may be rejected.

Applicant is found unsuitable at interview   There may be several reasons for rejection at this stage:

1 *Unsuitable as a volunteer:*

   ◆ Inform applicant then and there.

   ◆ Give reasons for not being selected—use discretion and ensure own safety. (Safety will include potential violence, sexual harassment, physical harm, or verbal abuse but also includes protection from false accusations.)

Thank them once again for the interest they have shown and for the time they have given.

2 *Unsuitable for their chosen area of work:*

   ◆ Give reasons for their not being selected—use discretion and ensure own safety.

   ◆ If appropriate, offer a review meeting in 6 months' time (e.g. the applicant has had a recent bereavement). It is a good idea to set a time for a review, as this will be interpreted as positive rather than as just 'a brush off'.

   ◆ Thank them once again for the interest they have shown and for the time they have given.

3 *No vacancies in the requested area:*

   ◆ Offer another work area or put on a waiting list for their chosen area—these offers may or may not be accepted; thank them once again for the interest they have shown and for the time they have given. VSMs may also direct the prospective volunteer to their local volunteer centre so that they may explore other possible volunteering opportunities.

Before potential volunteers leave after the informal interview ensure:

◆ Any paperwork or permission has been completed/sought (confidentiality statement, references); they have an opportunity to ask questions.

◆ They have clear information to take away:

- Contact details.
- Time and date of the next appointment.
- Details of the further 'selection hoops' and points of rejection.

A successful interview will result in the applicant progressing to the next stage of the selection process.

Induction

The details of an induction programme are discussed in Chapter 6. Here, induction is mentioned because it is a part of the selection process and needs to be completed successfully to enable further progression towards final selection. Induction can be a day, half a day, or series of sessions (e.g. weekly). All volunteers must attend induction. It will incorporate the basic legal requirements for insurance, health and safety, and confidentiality. Departmental induction in this chapter is referred to as part of probation.

Induction is the third point where an applicant may be rejected.

Unsuitability of an applicant or non-attendance

1 A person may interview well, but during induction as part of a group or team they may show poor interaction, communication, and team skills or may be very domineering, which may—depending on the role to be fulfilled—show the applicant to be unsuitable.

2 They may fail to attend some or the entire induction programme. The VSM should then:

◆ Contact the applicant—in writing, in person, or by phone.

◆ Set up an informal interview, if appropriate to:

- Discuss/consider mitigating circumstances.
- Discuss attitude/behaviour—use discretion and ensure own safety.
- Put further selection processes in place (e.g. review date).

Reject by letter or by telephone. If a volunteer has not completed the mandatory parts of their induction (e.g. health and safety, moving and handling, fire, confidentiality, etc.) in the timescales dictated by the organization, they cannot commence or continue work. The protocol for induction will vary among organizations (e.g. volunteers can attend their place of work four times before induction or they must receive induction within 6 weeks of commencing work, etc.). If the volunteer having been given every opportunity to attend the required sessions does not complete but still wishes to volunteer, then they will have to be re-interviewed and a risk assessment conducted as to their likelihood of attendance and completion of the mandatory requirements. Time and resources must be considered, as must the commitment and motivation of the individual. It could be a waste of time and money for both the applicant and the VSM.

Probationary period

The purpose of a probationary period is to give the new volunteer and the organization time to see if they have made the right choice. It is the time to set up suitable means of support and supervision and enables necessary training and assessment of skills and competency. It is a 'getting to know you' period.

This period is most often supervised by the managers/designated supervisors/team leaders in that work area rather than directly by the VSM. A planned departmental induction and competency criteria is agreed between the manager and volunteer. The criteria and induction package should have previously been agreed with the VSM adhering to the organization's induction strategy and established competency pathways.

During the probation period there may be some mandatory training to be undertaken (e.g. the use of hoists), but this time is also about being shown the 'ropes', being supervised, advised, and supported by a designated staff member (trained in mentorship/supervision) until the new volunteer applicant feels confident and competent and the mentor/team leader endorses this according to agreed criteria.

Throughout the probation period, the VSM is informed of the volunteer's progress by the line manager/team leader who will conduct regular reviews (formal or informal) with the volunteer. Any problems that the volunteer or staff experience should be discussed with the VSM, including any interpersonal or work conflicts, and a strategy for handling the situation to be decided between the VSM, the volunteer, and supervisory staff involved—protocols should be established for this. Sometimes, the practicalities of volunteers meeting with their mentors/supervisors can be difficult because of shifts, holidays, etc., and so their competency is not being properly assessed in agreed timescales or by the designated supervisors. If this situation persists, then the system used must be examined to see if it can be improved.

If the volunteer does not meet the probationary requirements by the end of the probation period, an extension can be granted in some circumstances if the staff in that area and the VSM agree that is the best way forward. If the volunteer is considered to be unsuitable or he/she is unhappy in that particular volunteer role, he/she may be offered an alternative work area or they may be asked to leave.

An interview at the end of a successful probation period is a good idea. This is usually conducted by the VSM or the team leader in that area of volunteer work. It marks the end of their probationary period, tells the volunteer what they have done well, where they can improve, but mainly it is a recognition of their commitment and welcomes them into the organization.

Dismissal or removal, at any time, of a volunteer from a work area should be authorized by the VSM after consultation with the staff and with the volunteer concerned. Procedures should be established for this.

Probation is the fourth point in the selection process where an applicant may be rejected.

Rejecting an applicant during / on completion of the probation period

If an applicant is rejected during or on completion of probation period:

◆ Inform the probationer—in person, at a planned interview and in writing.

◆ Give reasons for not being selected—use discretion and ensure own safety.

Rejection of an applicant at any stage in the process

The VSM should handle rejection firmly, fairly, and sensitively—think about how it feels to be rejected. When handling rejection:

◆ Temper with positive feedback.

◆ Suggest alternatives or ways forward.

◆ Highlight the positives of that individual.

◆ Maybe direct them towards another more suitable agency or towards some training that may be of benefit to them and to future applications.

◆ Try not to lie or couch the truth too heavily.

◆ Be constructive especially regarding criticism.

Bending the rules

From experience, a situation that the VSM and other staff may be confronted with is when a colleague, a manager, or a volunteer encourages the moving of a volunteer to another work area or brings in a new volunteer *without going through the normal volunteer selection system.*

This is unsafe practice and should be dealt with quickly and effectively but sensitively as well as firmly. Often, the individuals involved do not see the significance of their actions and can be quite shocked and upset by the reaction that their 'just trying to help' can cause.

> **Key issue:** If a selection policy and process are to be successful, the VSM should be a member of the senior management team and have their professional respect and support at all times. Breaches in the process usually point to the need for improved management and a review of policies.

Implementing the selection process

The selection standards and policies must be clear, robust, realistic—a true representation of the system in place—whilst reflecting the palliative care unit's philosophy of care, protection, and integrity. The documents defining selection and the policy underpinning it must be circulated and made freely available to all managers and staff, paid and unpaid. Education in the importance of the volunteer selection process may be included in the induction programme.

Selection of Trustees

In a charitable organization, such as many hospices and palliative care services, the most senior management is most often the Board of Trustees who carry ultimate legal responsibility for the running of the unit.

This section has been included here because, although the VSM may not be involved in Trustee selection, he/she they may well be involved in their induction.

Some Trustees will also work as volunteers within the hospice and an understanding of some of the issues around Trustees may be useful to highlight potential conflicts of interest and management problems.

The Trustees may often be the founding volunteers who helped to create the organization and defined its aims and objectives, decided the structure, policy, and philosophy, and often hold a legal and financial responsibility within the organization. As a result, they may have a strong feeling of ownership[4]. Within the framework they created, they made space for others like themselves—volunteers—partly in recognition of their monetary value and partly to allow others to gain the same sense of worth and achievement and satisfaction that they have experienced[3–5].

As an organization develops, the Trustees will change, as will the qualities and they skills they bring to the work. As time passes, fewer and fewer Trustees are the founding volunteers and more specific skills-based selection and recruitment may take place. The role of the Trustee changes as an organization grows and the role and responsibilities of Trustees must be clearly defined to ensure effective management and achievement of goals[4,5].

The eligibility criteria for Trustees will vary but will reflect the organization's constitution, 'company' and legal status. But there are some common features of a Board of Trustees:

♦ Trustees may have been selected from the organization's 'members' or 'friends' or its volunteer team.

♦ There may be 'time-served' criteria in place (e.g. 5 years as a volunteer, etc.).

♦ A Trustee position is usually a voluntary (i.e. unpaid) position.

Members of the Board of Trustees may have a financial obligation to the organization in case of a financial disaster. Trustees are usually elected on to the Board by other members of the company (some of whom are themselves volunteers) and will most likely have to produce and present their 'case' for election, providing personal and professional references and affidavits.

Trustees are selected because of their proven commitment to the organization and/or because they have particular relevant skills to offer (e.g., management, medical, accountancy, and legal skills, etc.).

In some organizations, there is the opportunity to 'co-opt' board members. The purpose of this is to ensure a comprehensive skill mix and equitable representation of views of interested parties. However, these 'volunteers' may have very little previous knowledge of the work of the organization and what knowledge they have may not be detailed.

It is desirable that all Trustees have an induction programme the extent of which will in part depend on their previous involvement with the organization and their knowledge base. In the United Kingdom, over 70 per cent of Trustees are from professional or intermediate occupations, and in 1995, 66 per cent did not receive any induction or training when they first became a Trustee[6].

It is suggested that new Trustees attend the mandatory induction that all other new paid staff and volunteers attend. In addition, there is a need for a Trustee-specific induction/education/training programme to explain the roles and responsibilities of Trustees and the board in relation to the hospice/palliative care service. When the individual needs of new Trustees are known, a programme of induction can be tailored for their needs.

Training of Trustees is discussed in Chapter 6 but a Trustee is usually in post for a minimum of 3 years (depending on the organization's constitution), and they can have a big impact on the organization's management and policy.

Trustees working as 'ordinary' volunteers

If someone wants to work in a 'hands on' volunteer role in addition to sitting on the Board of Trustees, are there any questions that need to be addressed?

◆ How will the other volunteers feel about this?

◆ Can this volunteer act in an appropriate manner in their role as a non-Trustee volunteer? Has the volunteer's attitude changed since becoming a Trustee and will/ does this cause conflict?

◆ How do the paid staff managing this volunteer feel?

◆ How do you, the VSM, feel? Do you feel you are able to manage this volunteer effectively?

Resentment and conflict can and do arise and the VSM must know how to tackle them.

Close relatives of salaried staff applying to be volunteers

A clear management policy is essential:

◆ What is the policy going to be and who decides it?

◆ Will it allow family members of paid staff to be accepted as volunteers or not? Will it allow family members of Board members/Trustees to become volunteers?

◆ What should an existing volunteer do when a family member becomes a paid member of staff or a Board member/Trustee? Should they discontinue volunteering (at least for the duration of the official appointment for Board members/Trustees)?

◆ How do you prevent nepotism—favouritism shown to family and friends?

The creation and adherence to this policy will once again be a reflection of the organization's senior management trust, support, and professional respect for the VSM.

Key issue: A clear policy needs to be in place about employing as a volunteer a close relative of a member of staff.

Documentation and data protection

Everything that the VSM does should be according to clear and realistic standards and policies that are reviewed and audited regularly to ensure best practice and regulated by relevant data protection legislation.

It is useful to sign/initial and date any written entries and maintain a record of the names and position held of those who have the right to write in the paper or computer files in the voluntary services office. The list will record the person's full name and signature and initials to help with the identification of entries.

Records should be appropriate, relevant and succinct—monitored, and audited regularly (quarterly, half-yearly, annually) and unnecessary data regularly removed. Confidentiality must be maintained with access to records (paper or computer), limited to designated users using a security system (locked cabinet/password-protected). It is advisable to keep paper records for a minimum of 6 to 8 years.

The volunteers must be aware of how and where their records are being kept. If these records are to be used for any mailing list, etc., by any one other than those in the organization, then permission must be sought of the individuals. Volunteers are entitled to request access to their records.

In conclusion, the selection of volunteers is exercising a legal and moral obligation to choose the best and most appropriate people for your organization— to guarantee quality and safety. A robust, effective, and equitable selection policy alongside a strong training and education strategy, will help to ensure that the common misunderstanding that 'voluntary' means 'amateur' does not persist.

Acknowledgement

The author wishes to acknowledge her indebtedness to Maggie Brain for her advice and help in preparing this chapter.

References

1 Davis Smith, J. (1997). Organising volunteers. In *Voluntary Matters—Management and Good Practice in the Voluntary Sector*, (eds. P. Palmer and E. Hoe), pp. 277–302. London, Directory of Social Change.

2 Plain English Campaign. www.plainenglish.co.uk

3 McCurley, S. and Lynch, R. (1998). *Essential Volunteer Management* (2nd edition). London, Directory of Social Change.

4 Hudson, M. (1999). *Managing without Profit—The Art of Managing Third Sector Organisations* (2nd edition). London, Penguin.

5 Ford, K. (1993). *The Effective Trustee. Part One: Roles and Responsibilities*. London, Directory of Social Change.

6 The Voluntary Sector National Training Organisation. (2000). *Draft Voluntary Sector Workforce Development Plan 2000*. www.nvco-vol.org.uk

Chapter 6

The training and education of volunteers

Sally-Ann Spencer-Gray

Purpose, aims, objectives, and outcomes

This chapter deals with training and education and although these terms are often used interchangeably they are subtly different.

Training is the act or process of teaching or learning a specified skill, especially by practice. This equips the individual for a specific task or role. The skills may be transferable but the outcome is quite discreet and measurable.

Education develops intellectual, moral, and social skills through systematic instruction and experience. It is a broader concept than training. It gives:

♦ Underlying knowledge

♦ Philosophy

♦ Understanding

♦ Skills that can be used in a variety of settings

The outcome is a deeper level of understanding that is diffuse, transferable, and not always easily measurable.

What do volunteers expect from their training and education?

It must be recognized that individuals have very different expectations of their volunteering experience. Some people will think of themselves as a 'professional volunteer', those whose 'job' to them is being a volunteer but most will consider themselves as 'being there to help', usually in their spare time.

Whilst all volunteers look for job and personal satisfaction from their volunteer experience, not everyone will want to take on responsibilities or 'develop'; but for some volunteers educational opportunities and career development may be very important.

Volunteering can be seen as:

♦ A stepping-stone to paid work or full-time education/training.

♦ An opportunity for free or reduced cost education and training.

♦ An opportunity to try something different—learn new skills/new experiences.

- An opportunity to consolidate prior learning/experience/skills.
- Providing a work record/references.
- A positive employment attribute, the public and potential employers see volunteers as trusted and caring people (especially volunteers working in a hospice or palliative care setting (i.e. working with the dying is often seen as the epitome of 'good work')).
- A negative employment attribute, where people believe volunteer work is for those who would not be considered suitable for paid employment.

The differences between individual expectations of the volunteer role together with previous educational experiences means that the training/education provided can be seen in different ways—a perk, threatening, a necessary evil, or as a great opportunity.

A good volunteer-selection process along with clearly defined educational opportunities—that are of direct benefit to patient care whilst not being a barrier or threat to potential volunteers—will help to avoid exploitation or misuse of your voluntary service as a 'training agency' and ensure the recruitment of committed volunteers.

Why is it necessary to train and educate volunteers?

One of the main purposes of the education of all staff and volunteers, is to ensure a *common minimum knowledge base* and a universal understanding of the philosophy, work, values, and role of the organization[1, 2].

Volunteer training/education is therefore provided to support patient care, to ensure standards of care and safe practice and to ensure appropriate public representation of the organization.

An introduction to the work of the voluntary service will ensure that the key principles of palliative care are understood[1:]

- Focus on quality of life.
- Whole-person approach.
- Care encompasses both the dying person and those who matter to that person.
- Patient autonomy and choice.
- Emphasis on open and sensitive communication.

It will ensure that no one is in any doubt as to what is expected of him/her regarding:

- Confidentiality.
- Professionalism.
- Maintaining the organization's good image and reputation.

It will also ensure:

- Appropriate information and skills to ensure safe and best practice are imparted.
- Which in turn will maintain quality and standard of work and care.
- Improved and on-going motivation.
- Enable personal development.
- Improve job satisfaction. Additional/further training/education will help an individual's professional and personal development but it is also only through the

training and education of staff that a service can grow and develop, its staff are a precious resource and should be nurtured. It must also be remembered that education is a two-way process, the organization can and must learn from its staff[3].

The three elements of volunteer training/education are statutory, mandatory, and voluntary: *Must, Should,* and *Could*

Statutory: *Must*

Required by law—local and national employment law, Health and Safety laws, etc. These include:

◆ All new volunteers.

◆ Updates to existing staff.

◆ Role change/development. The frequency and necessity of statutory training/ updates requirements must be made clear to each volunteer, failure to attend training/updates will mean that they cannot work or continue to work in that role. An example of statutory education/training is Moving and Handling (M&H)—a requisite of Health and Safety legislation and insurance. Every one *must* have comprehensive initial M&H training and then updates according to their role/risk (e.g. high, medium, low).

Mandatory: *Should*

Compulsory—a requirement determined by the organization. An organization will set minimum training standards/requirements that must be met in order for a volunteer to work in a specific role or area.

An example of mandatory education/training is the *induction* programme—this will be discussed in more detail later. In addition to a general induction there are three distinct working areas/categories to consider.

1 *Non-patient areas*

◆ Charity shops

◆ Donations transport—van drivers and assistants who collect donated items for resale in the charity shops

◆ Fund-raising

◆ Direct contact with the general public, which may include some contact with patients and/or relatives including bereaved relatives

◆ Home care

◆ Day care (day hospice)

◆ Inpatient area (bedded unit)

◆ Outpatient clinic (ambulatory clinic)

◆ Drivers for transport or patients

◆ Coffee bar or restaurant staff

◆ Bereavement support

- Reception
- Catering
- Housekeeping, etc.

2 *Patients and relatives contact areas*
All volunteers may work within patient areas and will have prolonged, regular contact with patients and/or relatives, including bereaved relatives.

3 *Working in a professional capacity* (see also Chapter 9)
This includes working unpaid as:

- Nurse
- Doctor
- Physiotherapist
- Hairdresser
- Complementary therapist, etc.
- Trustee/Board Member. These volunteers will need to produce evidence of relevant qualifications and registrations pertinent to their profession and may, in addition, need specific qualifications to work with patients with palliative care patients (e.g. lymphoedema massage).

An example of mapping training/education requirements is shown in Table 6.1.

Table 6.1 Volunteers: an example of training/education requirements

Induction	Non-patient areas	Patients and relatives contact areas	Working in a professional capacity
Customer service/ communication skills			
Finance/Cashier			
Fund-raising/Public liability/ health and safety			
Bereavement			
Clinical skills (e.g. feeding, bathing)			
Use of equipment (e.g. hoists)			
Drivers' training			
Basic first aid			
Food hygiene			
Disease information (e.g. Symptoms, nutrition)			
Task-specific training			
Trustee induction			
Trustee role-specific training			

Voluntary: *Could*

Chosen to undertake for professional and/or personal development not a required element:

+ To provide additional skills to enhance the volunteer role/job/experience.

+ Advanced learning (e.g. a counselling/or bereavement course), building on existing skills.

+ Unrelated to the volunteer role/job but will advance his/her personal skills and development (e.g. a computer course when working as a driver for patients, etc.). (Care must be taken regarding such payments in kind, and employment law— suggest volunteer pays for such training.)

Resources

Time, budget, appropriate trainers/educators, facilities, materials, and access

Before discussing in more detail the different programme options, there are a number of issues that require some discussion as they can affect the how, where, when, and why of the training/education provision.

Time: what time is available to dedicate to training?

This will depend on:

+ What the training is

+ Who is conducting it

+ Where they are conducting it; but must include an element of preparation time

+ What time are volunteers prepared to give?

+ Will they be put off if they have to attend numerous days of 'unnecessary' classes before they can even start to help?

This can be a particular problem with those working in non-patient areas (e.g. charity shops; they may not see the need or significance of patient care details and communication skills).

Budget: What budget has been made available for training?

+ Is there a training budget?

+ Is it a separate budget for volunteer training or is it part of a larger training budget?

+ Who administers the budget, and who says yes or no to different training requests?

+ Is any training charged?

+ Is there funding available for materials?

+ Is there funding available to buy in expertise?

+ Is there funding available to train people to teach or in subject specific skills (e.g. moving and handling)?

Appropriate trainers/educators: who does the training?

- Does the organization have an education department or some paid lecturers?
- Are you (the Voluntary Services Manager) expected to do the training?
- Do you have the skills/qualifications to train/educate?
- Who can help you?
- Do you have to buy in the expertise?
- Which courses need specialists to conduct them?
- Dose the introduction/induction programme need specialist input (e.g. Moving and Handling, Health and Safety to meet legal requirements or recognized standards)?
- Is it appropriate to ask volunteers to help to train/educate?
- What happens with 'on the job training'? Who and how are the supervisors/trainers in these areas designated? (See the *Delivery* section.)

Facilities and materials: do you have any dedicated training/ education rooms?

- Are they of adequate size—how many people can attend induction training at any one time is the room registered under Health and Safety to cater for this number.
- Do you have to share facilities with other departments and are these rooms conducive to learning?
- Are they air-conditioned/heated/ventilated?
- Are there enough chairs; are they comfortable?
- What equipment is available—screen, whiteboard, flip chart, video/DVD, etc.
- Do you have to share this equipment; is this a problem?
- Where are the rooms and toilets located do they have disabled access, is there public transport available?
- What refreshments are available—how often, are they free?
- Do you take the training out to sites (e.g. charity shops)?
- Do you have or need appropriate videos about the organization, fire regulations, etc.?
- Do you have access to presentation resources, e.g. powerpoint, to a flip chart, paper, and pens?
- Are you going to supply handouts, workbooks, or certificates?
- Who pays for printing and reprographics?

Access: routes to and through training and education (see Fig. 6.1)

- The existing volunteer will be given the opportunity for appraisal/assessment that will include a training needs analysis (TNA) that will identify new courses, updates, and refresher courses needed or wanted.
- Pathways and competencies—certain courses or areas of study/training when achieved in a pre-determined order will lead to a particular level of competency, which in turn can lead to taking on a specific role or level of responsibility (e.g. team leader).

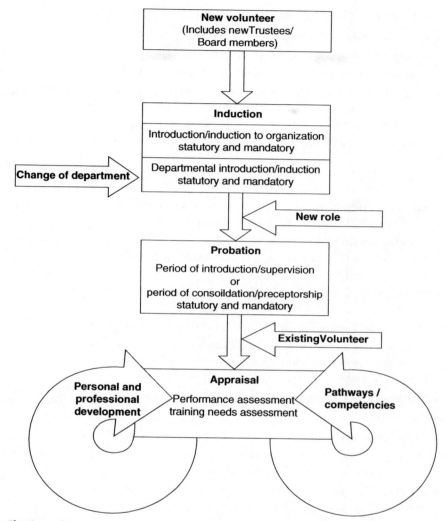

Fig. 6.1 Volunteers' access to and through training and education.

Planning

Purpose, content, and duration

For each course, lecture, pathway, and competency, the purpose, the content, the duration, and the assessment must be decided:

- Who is this course/lecture aimed at, will there be a mixture of volunteers, paid staff, and Board Members/Trustees?
- Will there be a cultural mix?

- Will it be a very mixed age group?
- What educational, literacy, and ability levels will be present?
- What are the audience's motivations for learning?
- What level is the course (i.e. basic/introductory, intermediate, advanced)?
- Is the course a registered academic course (i.e. registered with an external awarding body or is it a non-academic course certificated for attendance/achievement by the organization only)?
- Is it a stand-alone lecture/course or part of a competency pathway?
- What and how will it be assessed?

Course information document (CID)

It will help to write a course information document (CID) (or course information form or file—CIF). The CID will help you to identify:

- What the content of the course should be?
- What the learners should be able to do with the skills and knowledge they have (i.e. what tasks will it enable them to undertake)?
- Under what conditions should the learners be able to use their knowledge and skills to perform these tasks?
- How well do they need to perform the tasks and how will this be judged?

The CID will also be a resource to others but it will change—it is a working document and will reflect the information and understanding at that time.

In the CID state:

- The subject area experts (SAE) or subject matter experts (SME).
- The course leader.
- The teaching staff available.
- The target audience—who and how many—it is useful to state a maximum and minimum number needed for the course to be viable.
- The rationale—why is this course needed?
- The aims—general statements that indicate the purpose and general outcome of this learning.
- The objectives—more specific statements that will reflect the content.
- The learning outcomes—what you hope the attendees will be able to do by the end of the course. Indicative course content will state the:
  - Subjects to be covered and content of each session—must reflect the 'need' not what would be 'nice'.
  - Time allocated for this session.
  - Delivery method, the materials/facilities needed.
  - Method of assessment of completion/competency (e.g. attendance, number of times completed, etc.).

If particular videos, books, or exercises are used, they should be clearly stated here indicating their length, and copies of teaching materials and handouts should be available.

The experts may be paid staff or volunteers (i.e. the best people to help draw up the CID/CIF). Volunteer involvement will help to:

◆ Encourage ownership.

◆ Provide motivation to other volunteers.

◆ Keep the content relevant.

An example of successful volunteer involvement was in training drivers for the transport of patients.

> Experienced volunteer drivers were asked to help put together a short training session for new drivers, which they were delighted to do. In conjunction with the Voluntary Services Manager (VSM), they created an induction pack that included a training session, a 'task' checklist, and a buddy system for new drivers and they then went on to develop support/training sessions at regular intervals.

Involvement like this will highlight to volunteers their importance to the organization and respect of their views, it encourages communication between all staff, and helps team building[4, 5].

Having completed the CID it is good practice to circulate it to all interested parties, that is, other staff and volunteers involved in the relevant areas for their comments as to its content and format, asking:

◆ Is it realistic?

◆ Does it reflect what is needed?

◆ Is it achievable?

Volunteers' involvement and comment is very valuable and will often highlight views and issues previously overlooked.

Delivery

This section discusses theories on learning, skills, attitudes, and knowledge required for successful delivery and the methods employed.

How do we learn?

Training and education is not just about learning a specific skill, it is also an experience and should be a pleasant one. Learning is about change: a change in the way we see and think about the world around us and, ultimately, a change in how we interact with that world.

Volunteers working in palliative care will nearly all be adults and this fact should never be overlooked. When educating and training adults, their previous experience and knowledge must be acknowledged and valued[8], building on what they already know and can do.

We all employ what we learn in different ways:

◆ *Activists* are people who like to get on and get going straight away—they do not wait for instructions or read the manuals.

◆ *Reflective learners* like to sit back and think a while, perhaps watch someone else before having a go.

◆ *Theorizing learners* want to put things into a logical step-by-step order to make a clear straightforward picture out of a lot of complex information.

◆ *Experimental learners* want to experiment, they want to find new and more effective ways of doing things and they may take shortcuts.

In adult education, our teaching must be flexible and varied enough to accommodate and support all learning styles whilst still achieving the predetermined aims, objectives, and learning outcomes.

Skills, attitudes, and knowledge

What skills are needed to successfully deliver education and training to hospice volunteers? The following list of *Communication skills* has been developed from a list produced by Michael Meighan[4].

Active listening—awareness, understanding, and attention:

◆ Body language

◆ Non-verbal responses

◆ Appropriate verbal responses

◆ Summarizing

◆ Congruence

Effective presentation—to keep interest and provide clear information:

◆ Language—concise, non-jargon.

◆ Voice and eye contact—modulation and be inclusive. Remember, you are speaking to inform and impress with the content rather than with yourself the speaker.

◆ Use of equipment and aids—if you are using any audio or visual aids—you must be familiar with the content and the order.

◆ Look at content of audio visual aids—these should be relevant, concise and easy to read. Proof-read all written material. Good organization, preparation, and administration can make life a lot easier for yourself and others and shows efficiency and reliability. Ensure you, or those assisting you, have the knowledge required for the course:

• Self-awareness and self-knowledge—your own abilities, beliefs, prejudices, and values.

• Theories on learning.

• Structuring a programme—training needs, content, aims, and objectives, delivery, etc.

• People and behaviour, special needs, cultural, social, and religious needs.

- The effects of stress—in particular, the stresses that working in palliative care can create.
- Bereavement and loss theories.
- Group dynamics.
- Working with volunteers.
- The key principals of palliative care.
- Philosophy, purpose, work, and structure of the organization.
- Equity, equal opportunities.
- Appropriate national and international standards and legislation.

This is not a definitive list. In addition, every group you encounter is comprised of individuals. In effect, you are managing a group of individuals and you will need to have or develop the following:

- People skills—friendly approachable.
- Negotiating—respectful, adaptable, flexible.
- Motivation—positive, encouraging, enthusiastic.
- Problem-solving—helpful, caring, determined.
- Decision-making—assertive, confident, reliable.
- Selling—committed, realistic, observation—non-judgemental.
- Questioning.
- And at all times ensure confidentiality and keep a sense of humour.

Methods of delivery

Research and experience shows that we learn best through interaction and participation and retain 85 per cent of the information supplied, whereas through listening (in a lecture) we only retain 5 per cent of the information supplied.

Effective training/education will incorporate a number of delivery methods to ensure a varied programme that will make best use of resources and maintain interest. These will include:

- 'Show, tell, and do'.
- Didactic—lectures.
- Discussion.
- Role-play.
- Group work. Group work helps 'break the ice'; it gets people talking to each other and working together and, if you are doing more than one group work exercise, it is useful to get the people to swap around to form different groups each time—so making them talk and work with a different set of people.
- 'Show, tell, and do'[5]:
  - Shown either through the use of models or diagrams or by the teacher performing the task.

- Told the information.
- Doing—the student has a go. Most often the telling and showing go together—
'doing' is not always possible.

◆ *Didactic*, lectures are not very interactive and should be kept short and interspersed with activities. Support with written information.

◆ *Discussion* can work well but the group needs to 'gel' for this to work best. Discussion can be useful when looking at issues around confidentiality and boundaries.

◆ *Role-play* is very useful especially for communication skills but you will find that nobody (or very few) will want to take part—will work best with a group who have got to know each other a little.

Training/education programmes

The full training and education programme that is available to volunteers through your organization may be vast and there is not the space here to discuss the different variations that could be made available. However, it is worth considering what your organization's stance is regarding education and training as this attitude or commitment will determine what is provided, at what level, and for what purpose.

A full range of training/education will include the basics for advanced courses, formal or informal learning, leading to a certificate of attendance, competency to perform a specific task, or even a local or national qualification or certification. The training/education opportunities may be provided 'in house' but will also take advantage of external resources, including conferences, association/society, and committee membership. Volunteers should also be included in any organizational representation (e.g. ethics committees, awareness campaigns, etc.).

The learning experience should always be a positive one. One must not assume that an adult learner is an experienced learner; often, their last learning experience was many years ago at school and they may feel they have 'got out of the habit' or feel threatened just by the thought it. We have all had a bad education experience at some time in our lives (usually school) and these along with lack of motivation and boredom can be barriers to learning.

Learning must be recognized as an active process—it is interaction with a purpose.

Induction

A good induction is neither complex nor costly. It requires a clear and explicit process and good communication[6].

Volunteer introduction/induction will be based around thanks and gratitude and around the 'must know', 'should know', and 'could know' of a new job/environment. All those engaged in the learning must feel valued, respected as an individual, needed, and welcomed—they are going to be an asset and complementary to the high-quality service already provided.

Induction needs to be professionally informal—reflecting the ambience, hospitality, and atmosphere of the organization and its care. It must be a well-planned programme using good techniques. The involvement of different staff members in the delivery adds variety but also demonstrates team working and some friendly interdisciplinary banter helps to create a relaxed and friendly atmosphere. By employing a combination of 'teaching' staff—some of whom are clinical staff, and not primarily educationalists, can subliminally communicate an amazing number of messages[7, 8].

The induction programme

The induction programme (it can also be called 'orientation') will include[7, 8]:

◆ Cause or organization orientation

◆ System orientation

◆ Social orientation: direction and bearings—finding one's way

Cause or organization orientation: an introduction to the work of the organization

This includes:

◆ History

◆ Description of the cause

◆ The client group

◆ Mission statement

◆ Values and philosophy

◆ Programmes and services

◆ Future plans

This will enable a conscious decision, an emotional and intellectual commitment to the basic purpose of the organization.

System orientation: an introduction to the organizational systems

This includes the volunteer management system. Use 'What would I like to know?' to draw up a list that includes:

◆ The structure (management, hierarchy).

◆ Funding and fund-raising.

◆ Volunteer involvement in the organization:

  • Roles

  • Responsibilities

  • Reporting/management

  • Policies and procedure

◆ Facilities and equipment.

◆ Key activities. Providing organizational context, where the volunteer fits in and where particular roles fit into the whole. It also enables the volunteer to understand the organization and so be an effective communicator on behalf of the organization.

Social orientation: introduction to the organization's social community

This includes the staff, trustees, other volunteers—where the individual volunteer fits in. Some of this will take place as part of the departmental induction but the basics will be covered in the organizational induction:

- Introduction to colleagues.
- Introduction to support systems and to supervisors/mentors.
- Highlighting the benefits of volunteering for the individual.
- Looking at the opportunities available for growth and development.
- Reinforcing the value of their contribution.

An *accompanying written introduction pack* will include the organization's mission statement, philosophy, volunteering policy, moving and handling, health, safety, and fire policies (as bulleted lists) and contact information.

The generic induction you choose may be short and basic, or longer and more detailed and, therefore, will affect the content of any departmental induction.

Departmental induction

This can be seen as:

- Part of the probation period.
- Including mandatory training.
- Specific to the needs of the department.
- Devised between the manager and the volunteer.
- Individual to that volunteer based on the job-specification for that role.

Task-specific training/education

Those topics identified as 'task-specific' indicate that this is training to a level of competency in a specific task (e.g. patient feeding, using hoists). There will also be either a preceptorship (period of teaching or instruction) or a supervised period, whereby an individual will introduce the use of his/her skills clinically in a measured way. Each task will have minimum supervisory criteria associated with the competency. This supervisory/preceptorship period, or aspects of this period, can be increased to meet individual needs, at the request of the volunteer or their supervisor, to ensure that both parties feel confident and secure.

The 'qualified staff' involved in the procedure (this may include volunteers) and current legislation will determine the competencies of a task. Feedback from volunteers should be incorporated into decision making—often, the volunteers are the best people to be involved in drawing up training and competency initiatives.

Probation

Each volunteer will be allocated a mentor/supervisor by the manager of that department with whom they will meet regularly. It will be the responsibility of *both people* in this relationship not only to draw up and agree a probationary period timetable to include statutory and mandatory education and training, but also to ensure that these agreed goals are supported and met. A checklist of these criteria can be held by both parties and used to ensure that the criteria are met (checked and signed) and that minimum time scales are adhered to (see Appendices).

The responsibility of successful completion of the probationary period lies with both parties. The mentor/supervisor relationship continues after probation and forms the basis for continued assessment and appraisal.

Evaluation

In order to ensure that your course is on track, you need to evaluate it. Evaluation will involve feedback from the volunteers who will be given the opportunity to comment on the quality, the content, the delivery, and the usefulness of the course. At the end of each course an evaluation form should be completed by all attendees, allowing comment on individual elements of the course and on the course overall.

Evaluation of outcomes will come from volunteer feedback but also through evaluation of the volunteer's knowledge and work once they are in a department via their mentor/supervisor/manager.

Some of the outcomes from induction or other courses are not going to be instantly apparent immediately after a course and will only become evident in time and after some experience. The mentorship, supervision, and preceptorship of volunteers that form part of their probation should provide feedback on how much they have taken on from the courses they have attended and how well they integrate that to their practice. This gives information on the progress of the volunteer but also to some extent, on the usefulness of the content and effectiveness of the delivery of a course. The volunteer at regular mentor/supervisor meetings will be asked to comment regarding their induction and further training.

All feedback should be treated seriously and a method of collation and audit of this information should be in place. Similar suggestions received independently from a number of people, paid staff, or volunteers should be acted on—which may mean adjustment to the content or delivery or assessment associated with a course. (See Fig. 6.2.)

Standard setting and audit

This enables the value, content, and outcomes of courses, competencies, and pathways to be determined, tested, and changed if necessary. It will also allow for changes in legislation, approach, and the recommendations of research. The setting of standards enables audit of quality and effectiveness and provides a minimum standard framework to adhere to.

Assessment

Most people hate the idea of assessment and are often intimidated by the idea that they are to be 'tested', but somewhere along the line a judgement has to be made as to the suitability of the volunteer to a job or environment.

Assessment recognizes achievement, identifies goals, and motivates.

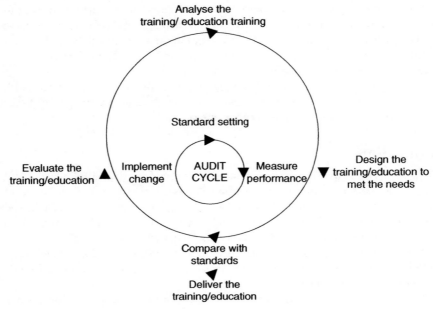

Fig. 6.2 The training and audit cycle[4].

Usually, volunteer assessment is seen as informal and non-threatening but some volunteers prefer a more formal approach, so assessment of volunteers needs to be flexible and to meet the needs of the organization and of the volunteer. All organizations do some form of assessment.

Appraisal

Most organizations will have an appraisal scheme. Appraisal is a support mechanism and should not be used as a route for punishment. Volunteers' formal use of the appraisal scheme is usually optional: some may like to have formal feedback on their performance and the opportunity to put a training needs analysis together, as previously discussed. Others feel threatened by this perceived 'judging' of their performance and prefer a more informal approach.

Continuous assessment is important for both the organization and the volunteer:

◆ Encourages volunteer involvement and motivation.

◆ Monitors performance and provides feedback on progress.

◆ Helps to ensure quality and maintenance of standards.

◆ Helps in shaping the volunteers future learning scheme—training needs analysis. All assessments/interactions must be documented this will be especially important at times of conflict or discipline. Volunteers, like paid staff, are subject to and protected by the disciplinary and grievance procedures and legislation relevant to your organization.

The manager/team leader will give appropriate feedback to the VSM when necessary—usually when there is a problem.

Training records

The holding of statutory, mandatory, and individual training records may be the responsibility of the VSM, the education/training department or officer, or the volunteer himself/herself.

The planning, delivery, evaluation, and audit of the education/training provided can be the responsibility of the VSM or a designated education/training staff member or department.

Whatever system is in place or you choose to adopt, the following points are essential:

- Clearly state who is responsible for what—induction, probation, training, and appraisal.
- The staff involved in education, appraisal, supervision, mentorship, and preceptorship are suitably trained and supervised.
- Someone takes on the responsibility of holding the volunteer training records and ensures notification of statutory and mandatory updates.
- The written minimum standards for induction/probation are being met and course content and competencies meet with local and national guidelines, insurance, and Health and Safety legislation.
- There is a reporting mechanism for problems/grievances.
- Evaluation is regularly conducted and the results utilized.

Training and education of Trustees

As stated in Chapter 5 on the selection of volunteers, Trustees are usually selected because of their proven commitment to the organization and/or because they have particular relevant skills to offer (e.g. management, medical knowledge, accountancy skills, etc.). Some Trustees will therefore be new to your organization and may have very little previous knowledge of the its work.

The responsibility for Trustees' education and training can vary from organization to organization. It may well be the responsibility of the VSM and/or the education officer/department especially where it overlaps with established courses, or it may be considered the sole responsibility of the Board and senior management.

It is preferable that some of the Trustees' induction would be conducted alongside other staff and volunteers to encourage openness, understanding, and team working. It is also advisable that any further educational requirements are devised/developed with educational staff/department input/advice.

Trustee induction should be based around:

- Cause or organization orientation
- System orientation
- Social orientation

What do Trustees need in their induction?

In addition to attending the organization's normal introduction/induction, an annual induction for new Board Members should be instigated. It must be acknowledged that some organizations will have insufficient new Trustees at any one time to justify running an annual induction session and so alternative induction programmes should be devised, for example, a workbook and individual sessions, or working with other similar organizations to provide a local or regional resource[6].

Trustee-specific induction information

This comprises the following:

◆ The organization's constitution.

◆ The purpose and functions of the Board of Trustees—terms of reference for the Board and committees—powers and rules of governance.

◆ Specific Trustee roles and responsibilities—chair, vice chair, treasurer, other officers, etc., and as ambassador/representative of the organization to the public—codes of conduct.

◆ Confidentiality—particular responsibilities regarding Board/organizational activities.

◆ Boundaries—to also include work of the Board and work of the managers.

◆ Trustees' liabilities and protection.

◆ Management philosophy and methodology—basic management options and methodology, adopted by the organization, members/roles of the management team, staffing policy, etc.

◆ Clinical audit, clinical governance, and quality standards.

◆ Supervision/mentorship, grievance, and disciplinary procedures/policies.

◆ Funding/financial management.

◆ The law—constitution and local, national, and international legislation.

◆ Further education opportunities.

◆ Health and Safety responsibilities of the Trustees.

Specific Trustee skills/education/training

These skills include:

◆ Presentation skills.

◆ Chair—responsibilities and duties.

◆ Vice Chair—responsibilities and duties.

◆ Meetings—committee process and purpose.

◆ Treasurer—finance/accounting information/skills (identified as the most frequently occurring knowledge gap for Trustees)[9]. The Board of an organization is a coalition of people from a variety of backgrounds who must work together; they will provide leadership and must add value and be of benefit to the organization.

A Trustee/Board Member should at all times uphold the Nolan Committee's seven principles of public life[10]:

1 Selflessness
2 Integrity
3 Objectivity
4 Accountability
5 Openness
6 Honesty
7 Leadership

The Nolan Committee also recognizes the need to promote and reinforce standards of conduct of all those engaged in public life through guidance and training, including induction training.

Acknowledgement

The author wishes to acknowledge her indebtedness to Maggie Brain for her advice and help in preparing this chapter.

Appendix 1

Orientation checklist—Page 1

The following example is indicative only. The first date refers to the date the mentor shows/discusses the item. The volunteer's initials and date confirm that they have received and understood the information.

	Date	Mentor's initials	Date	Volunteer's Initials
Volunteer's name:				
Mentor's name:				
Date attended induction:				
Date of first attendance in department:				
Introduced to the staff: who's who				
Shown department layout				
Shown emergency exits				
Shown the location of fire alarm points				
Discussed their role in case of fire				
Shown how to use the telephone system				
How and who to telephone in case of an emergency				
Importance and procedure of taking accurate messages				
Moving and handling procedures				
Mentor, probation, and appraisal systems				
Confidentiality (statement signed)				
Boundaries and reporting mechanisms				
'Role description' discussed				

Orientation checklist—Page 2

Summary of initial meeting with the volunteer discussing relevant skills, attributes, interests, and abilities the volunteer feels they can offer to the department:

Date: Mentor's signature:

Date: Volunteer's signature:

Please identify any areas of concerns or perceived problems:

Date: Mentor's signature:

Date: Volunteer's signature:

Please identify any particular support or special needs required:

Date: Mentor's signature:

Date: Volunteer's signature:

What additional mandatory training has been identified?

Date: Mentor's signature:

Date: Volunteer's signature:

Appendix 2

Mentor/supervision record—Page 1

Volunteer's name:

Mentor's name:

Length of probationary period (e.g. 3 months):

Date probationary period begins:

Date probationary period will end:

Agreed frequency of review/supervision meetings
(e.g. weekly for 4 weeks and then fortnightly)

Review frequency at end of probation period:

Date:

Mentor's signature: Volunteer's signature:

Was the probation period completed successfully? YES/NO

If NO please briefly state reasons and action here:

Review of frequency of mentor/supervision meetings, date:

Please state changes to the schedule here:

Date of first annual appraisal (if requested):

Mentor/supervision record—Page 2

Date of mentor/ supervision meeting	Mentor's initials	Volunteer's initials	Comments

Appendix 3

Probation checklist—Page 1

Volunteer's name (V): Mentor/supervisor's name (M):Date probation begins: Date probation ends: Following is a list of agreed competencies to be completed during the probationary period.

Task details: (e.g. use of hoist) Agreed competency pathway: e.g. 30-min training session with mentor, observe use 1, assisted in use 1, supervised use 2. To be completed by:

Training M V   Observed M V   Assisted M V   Supervised M V   Supervised M V

Date

Volunteer feels confident and is deemed competent, date:

Mentor's signature: Volunteer's signature:

Task details: Agreed competency pathway: To be completed by:

Training M V   Observed M V   Assisted M V   Supervised M V   Supervised M V

Date

Volunteer feels confident and is deemed competent, date:

Mentor's signature: Volunteer's signature:

Probation checklist—Page 2

End of probationary period review meeting, date: Was probation period successfully completed? YES/NO

If NO please state reasons and agreed action here:

If YES were any further education/training needs identified?

Date

Mentor's signature: Volunteer's signature:

References

1 National Council for Hospice and Specialist Palliative Care Services (NCHSPC). (1996). *Education in Palliative Care*. London, NCHSPC.

2 National Council for Hospice and Specialist Palliative Care Services (NCHSPC). (1997). *Making Palliative Care Better: Quality Improvement, Multiprofessional Audit and Standards*. Occasional Paper 12. Glickman M/Working Party on Standards. London, NCHSPC.

3 Hudson, M. (1999). *Managing without Profit—The Art of Managing Third Sector Organizations* (2nd edition). London, Penguin.

4 Meighan, M. (1995). *How to Design and Deliver Induction Training Programmes* (2nd edition). London, Kogan Page.

5 Forsyth, I., Joliffe, A., and Stevens, D. (1999). Delivering a course—Practical strategies for teachers. In *Lecturers and Trainers* (2nd edition). London, Kogan Page.

6 The Ford Partnership and Help the Hospices. (2000). *The Trustee Induction Pack— The Twenty-Minute Guide to Being a Hospice Trustee*. London, Help the Hospices.

7 McCurley, S. and Lynch, R. (1998). *Essential Volunteer Management* (2nd edition). London, Directory of Social Change.

8 Smith, J. D. (1997). Organising Volunteers. In *Voluntary Matters—Management and Good Practice in the Voluntary Sector*, (ed. P Palmer and E Hoe), pp. 277–302. London, Directory of Social Change.

9 The Voluntary Sector National Training Organisation. (2000). *Draft Voluntary Sector Workforce Development Plan 2000*. http://www.nvco-vol.org.uk

10 Her Majesty's Stationery Office (HMSO). (1995). *The Nolan Committee's First Report on Standards in Public Life*. London, HMSO.

Chapter 7

The support of volunteers

Gill Hamilton

Hospices and palliative care units, especially in the United Kingdom, often have large volunteer teams that provide additional support to the staff and patients and enhance the environment of the organization. These individuals come to offer their time and skills for a variety of reasons and their level of commitment and dedication is very special. Whoever they are, whatever they do, however long they work for the palliative care service, they need to receive appropriate support. This chapter will address this challenge.

It is important that volunteers are fulfilled in their role and that they enjoy both the experience and their involvement with the organization, not least because this will encourage them to stay with the organization for some time. As highlighted in Chapter 3, the introduction of a voluntary service has to be based on a clearly defined plan, policy, and budget which clearly details how the service will be managed and how volunteers will be managed, from the first interview of the prospective volunteers to the time they leave the service.

This chapter will suggest ways in which volunteers may be supported during their time within the organization. The main text will take the 'career' of the volunteer from beginning to end, discussing at each stage how this support might be delivered. As support and training are closely liked, this chapter will touch on areas that are discussed in more depth in Chapter 6. However, it is important to consider training and education from the standpoint of the support strategy that is in place for volunteers.

Introducing a voluntary service

Volunteer policy

The support of volunteers can begin even before they present themselves for interview by ensuring that a volunteer policy is in place[1]. This sets out how the organization intends to manage, protect, and support their volunteers during their time with the hospice. It is considered to be best practice to have a volunteer policy that covers the care, support, and supervision necessary to ensure a happy, satisfied volunteer group. But it is not only an important document for the volunteers; outside agencies, for example, those intending to provide funds, may also want to know that such a document is in place. A volunteer policy is a strong statement that shows an organization is clear about why it wants to involve volunteers.

Support at the interview stage

It is crucial that the interview and selection process for volunteers is effective for the organization and the individuals concerned. Supporting a volunteer should begin here at this first stage of their application to join the service. Details of good and effective interviews are covered in Chapter 5, but here we need to note not how to conduct an effective interview, but why it is so important. Supporting volunteers at the interview stage is important to ensure the hospice strikes the right balance between being formal and informal. Hospices need to interview volunteers to ensure, amongst other things, the volunteer is emotionally able to cope with their role and the environment. Volunteers also need to know that the hospice is right for them—that it is the place they want to contribute their time and skills to. Nevertheless we should not forget that, volunteering is not paid work and interviews can make it look a lot like it is. We also know that formality can deter volunteers for whom interviews are a daunting prospect. The Voluntary Services Manager (VSM) therefore has a role to play in guiding volunteers through the interview process, ensuring procedures are adhered to, but also ensuring that the hospice is a welcoming environment for volunteers.

Support before the first time on duty

As discussed in Chapter 6, some organizations prefer their new volunteers to attend an induction/ orientation/education course before they start their duties. These valuable courses can be especially useful in areas where the volunteer is involved as a one-to-one buddy with a client or patient. In particular, these sorts of tasks require volunteers to have information, help, and support before starting their duties.

There are both advantages and disadvantages of providing courses before a volunteer starts.

Advantages:

◆ Volunteers may feel better prepared and more comfortable to come into the unit to carry out their tasks.

◆ Volunteers will meet other new volunteers at the course.

They may have had a chance at the course to listen to and speak to an experienced volunteer. This can be a very positive experience to new volunteers.

Disadvantages:

◆ Such courses can only be organized on a regular basis every 4 to 6 months because staff members are involved, or because courses can only be run when 'enough' new volunteers have been recruited to make a course viable. If volunteers have to wait until completing a course before starting regular duties, such delays can result in the volunteer becoming impatient and seeking another organization.

◆ Volunteers may feel less comfortable about helping in palliative care because they only hear about but do not yet have the opportunity to experience the special ambience that all units have.

◆ The success of the course depends considerably on the content and those who deliver it in order to maintain the interest of the new volunteers before they have experienced the area for themselves.

◆ Volunteers who have not had previous experience of courses or education sessions may be put off because they perceive it as too formal an approach. All they wish to do is give their time to the hospice.

◆ Volunteers who have previous experience of courses, seminars, and education sessions during their working life may not want to have to take part in these kinds of meetings in order to become a volunteer.

Providing courses within 6 months of the new volunteer starting duty also has its advantages and disadvantages.

Advantages:

The new volunteer has come to know the unit and some of the staff and feels comfortable about coming in to the course. They:

◆ Meet other new volunteers who have just joined.

◆ Have not had to wait to get started on their duties. Motivation is very important, and it is good for new volunteers to start working as soon as possible.

◆ Have some knowledge of the work and come with questions to the sessions and an eagerness to learn more about palliative care.

Disadvantages:

◆ They may have not had the knowledge or confidence gained from a course to support the staff effectively even though their on-duty training has been carried out.

◆ They have not developed their awareness and understanding of palliative care through the course before starting in their role. However the courses are offered, they are essential to develop the knowledge, interest, and awareness of new volunteers.

Support on the first day of duty

Support at this stage is primarily about being warmly welcomed into the unit preferably by someone the new volunteer has already met, usually the VSM. The volunteer should have some background reading about the hospice before coming in for the first time. This helps with understanding palliative care and how the particular unit cares for its patients and families. The next important step is to give them a short induction/orientation programme as covered in Chapter 6.

Volunteers come in with great enthusiasm to start their duty but the first visit can be a daunting time for some new volunteers who may be anxious about it for many reasons, some of which may include concerns such as:

◆ Will it be a sad place?

◆ Who will I be working with and will I like them?

◆ How will I feel when I go through these doors into the ward area?

◆ Will I manage to control my emotions if I see unexpectedly someone I know?

◆ Can I cope with what is expected of me?

◆ Will there be help nearby if I have a problem?

◆ Am I at risk from these hospital infections I hear about?

- What will I get out of this commitment of time?
- Will I find satisfaction in this role?
- Do I really have the skills that are needed in this area of palliative care?

All of these areas of concern need to be addressed at the induction programme by the VSM and are most likely to be answered after the probationary period has been completed as discussed in the following paragraphs. It is likely that since the successful interview, the new volunteer has had time to think about the task taken on and will need reassurance at this early stage.

The probationary period

The new volunteers will know before they start that a probationary period is a necessary part of the initial phase of their time with the organization. This support mechanism should be written into the volunteer policy and should apply to all volunteers no matter what area they have chosen to help the organization. This period should extend over the first 3 or 4 months. It is a most important time because it is often found that people who volunteer for a palliative care organization do not really know how they will react to the environment.

At the end of this probationary period, in some organizations, a volunteer agreement will be discussed and signed by both the VSM and the volunteer. Organizations can be reluctant to have such agreements because of fears of implying a contract with the volunteer (see Chapter 8 on legal aspects of volunteering). However, as long as these avoid the language of contracts and obligations, they can be very beneficial. The agreement should set out how expenses will be paid and what supervision and training is available. The agreement should be couched in terms of hopes and understandings and make clear that no obligations are placed on the volunteer.[1] The end of the probationary period also gives the volunteer an opportunity to discuss aspects of their duties that have not been easy for them. Of course, volunteers should always be informed of the 'open door' policy of the volunteer services office. This gives them freedom at any time to bring anxieties or questions to the attention of the volunteer office staff in the early days.

The commonest problems volunteers mention at this stage are:

- *Difficulties with the volunteer(s) with whom they share duty.* One solution may be to try to find another 'slot' in the timetable for them or to try to resolve the difficulties.
- *The timing is difficult for them.* Offer another duty time or another duty at a more convenient time.
- *The duty is suitable in summer but not in winter because of dark evenings.* Offer a day-time slot if possible or arrange transport home in winter. Seasonal volunteers can be awkward to manage unless they are prepared each time they go 'on sabbatical' to join a new area or duty on their return.

---

[1] Volunteering England provides very good advice on these; guidance can be found at http://www.volunteering.org.uk/Resources/goodpracticebank/Core+Themes/volunteerpolicies/volunteeragreements.htm

- *The cash till too awkward to handle.* Offer another duty. (This is an example of any duty that the volunteer can't adapt to; the solution is not to look on the volunteer as unsuitable, but to try to find another role.)

- *The duty is uninteresting. They need to be kept busy and the duty can be dull at times.* Again, offer another duty at a busier time.

- *Lacking the same enthusiasm or motivation with which they applied to help.* It may be that the organization is not for them. They must be given the chance to share this with the VSM and move to another organization if nothing can be done to address the issue. On the other hand, VSMs also need to recognize that motivations can change and may want to explore what those new motivations are and explore with the volunteer how these may be met by volunteering with the hospice.

The VSM must give time and effort to this part of the individual support of new volunteers. It is crucial that in such a caring environment, the volunteers feel that they themselves are cared for. They may find themselves unable to offer good care if their expectations as a volunteer are not fulfilled.

The new volunteer must know where to find help, how to contact the person in charge of their area, and at all times to feel able to contact staff from the volunteer office. The induction session is important in highlighting this information. This support helps to make the new volunteer feel that they are part of the team, reduces anxiety, and gives a good impression of the care and support to come in the months, possibly years ahead as they help in the organization.

The first spell of duty will involve training for the specific task the volunteer has undertaken. This training is often delivered by an experienced volunteer as outlined in Chapter 6.

On the day of their first duty after training, the new volunteer should not be left alone but be accompanied by an experienced volunteer for support and advice. Most volunteers enjoy the company of others and for some this can be the main motivation for applying to become a volunteer. Duties that isolate volunteers in a room or area where there is little contact with other people may be difficult to sustain. Those who take on such duties are likely to need more support and attention than those who work together in a small team on a regular basis.

Support through training, documentation, and education sessions

The details of training very much depend on the work the volunteer will do. How much they need and for how long are matters for each organization to evaluate. A good guide would be that the closer a volunteer is likely to be to patients or relatives, and especially if they are actually working with patients, then the more rigorous the training they will need.

One method of supporting a volunteer who is interested in contact with patients is to allow the volunteer to spend at least 6 months carrying out more routine tasks, such as in the coffee shop or flower room, before they move into patient care. This gives the volunteer time to get to know and understand the organization and how it operates and consequently gain confidence. It also gives the VSM and staff in the area concerned time to get to know the volunteer. This helps with selecting the appropriate volunteers for those teams that offer duties that involve working closely with patients.

Induction pack for volunteers

Providing a new volunteer with documentation in the form of an induction pack is an essential means of early support. Much information is given in the first phase of joining the volunteer service, and it is unlikely that most volunteers will retain everything that is explained to them. Giving them written information about their duty is most useful and serves as a reference for them when queries do arise.

This induction pack can contain items such as:

◆ A letter of welcome.

◆ A brief history of the hospice and the services it offers.

◆ A floor plan of the unit.

◆ Information on health and safety.

◆ A list of the many roles undertaken by volunteers in the palliative care service.

◆ Guidelines for the particular role the volunteer is being asked to undertake.

◆ Information about the processes in place for continuing support for volunteers (e.g. details of the probationary period, the first anniversary review, long-service medals/badges given to volunteers).

◆ The volunteer agreement and what it contains where this is in place.

◆ Emergency procedures in the event of fire and accident.

◆ A copy of the volunteer policy.

◆ An illustrated guide to the staff uniforms to help them identify staff categories, if appropriate.

Ongoing training and update sessions

Continuing education and update sessions are an essential component of support. They keep the volunteers up–to-date with developments of the organization and its environment and help them to maintain a sense of confidence in what they are doing.

Update sessions are opportunities for volunteers to learn more about the hospice/palliative care service, to hear about new developments, to get information about changed routines and to meet new members of staff. They are invaluable for many reasons, for example they may:

◆ Help the volunteers to feel valued and part of the bigger team, as they respond well to having staff explain and talk to them about the staff needs.

◆ Provide a means of communication with staff. This contact should be encouraged in these sessions as it helps greatly with relationships between staff and volunteers, which is vital for happy, productive teamwork.

◆ Give volunteers an opportunity to talk to staff and ask questions regarding their duties. Occasionally, volunteers might make suggestions which will, ultimately, help not only the staff and volunteers working alongside them but also the patients.

It cannot be emphasized enough that members of staff have a key role to play in helping volunteers to remain motivated and satisfied to stay in their roles for long periods of time. Working with and caring for volunteers should be integral in to staff training and should be monitored carefully. Volunteers should be acknowledged, recognized, and valued when they are in the hospice and thanked regularly by the staff.

Ongoing support

The organization that is supported by volunteers in turn requires to support them in a range of ways as they go about their duties. Volunteers should not only be shown how much they are appreciated, they should know of the many things that have been put in place for them as well as for the staff. This may include:

◆ Insurance. They should be reassured that there is adequate cover to protect them and the organization.

◆ Out-of-pocket expenses. On joining the service, volunteers should be advised that these are available to ensure that anyone who feels that they are unable to afford to come in to help will not be disadvantaged. Expenses are usually paid in arrears on presentation of a receipt.

◆ First anniversary of joining the volunteer service. On this anniversary, no matter how often the VSM has seen the volunteers in the preceding year, it is good practice to meet with the volunteers to thank them for their year's effort and to ask if they have any ideas, suggestions, or problems to discuss. These opportunities to be with a volunteer and listen to their comments are of great value and again reaffirms that they are part of a caring supportive team.

◆ Annual informal meetings. Ideally, the VSM should meet each volunteer, not only on the first anniversary, but on an annual basis. However, in most palliative care units and hospices, where volunteer numbers are large, this is not always possible or practicable. Even if such meetings are less frequent, say every 2 or 3 years, they are valuable for both the volunteer and the VSM.

◆ Team meetings and update education sessions as described above are important ways of bringing volunteers together.

◆ Social events. There is no doubt that such events are occasions when volunteers who might not otherwise see each other can do so in relaxed informal settings. However, much thought needs to be given to them and their cost. Many hospices and some palliative care units are run on a charitable basis and care must be taken, when organizing events for volunteers or rewarding them for their efforts. Volunteers generally do not wish the organization to spend money on them to say 'thank you' and so this aspect of support needs to be sensitively handled. Many units find the best times to run them are at Christmas or during 'Volunteer's Week' (UK).

◆ Long-service awards. Many units offer their volunteers some sort of reward, be it a certificate or badge which they can wear when on duty. The first is usually awarded after 5 years' service, then every 5 years thereafter. Each period of 5 years is marked either by a different brooch or a 'bar' to the medal. This is usually very acceptable to volunteers, and if the award is a special badge, they wear it with pride and indeed look forward to receiving it at a modest social occasion where the presentation is made by a the Chairman of the Trustees or a local dignitary.

◆ Special events. Some palliative care units and hospices recognize special birthdays, anniversaries, and the retirement dates of retired volunteers by sending cards or even flowers. Obviously, this recognition usually depends on the time the volunteer was with the organization and can be formally set out in the volunteer staff policy.

◆ Christmas and festivals. Depending on whatever are the local festivals and holidays such as Christmas, Passover, and New Year, volunteers can be sent a card or invited to a social event to mark these occasions.

◆ Cards or flowers. Volunteers who experience illness or bereavement may be sent a card or flowers from the volunteer office. A visit from a member of the volunteer office staff may also be considered. This kind of recognition during difficult times is always much appreciated.

◆ Voluntary services newsletter. This is an excellent way of communicating with volunteers as they can be kept abreast of any new developments, such as new members of staff, additions to the buildings, and any news with particular relevance to the volunteer service itself. It may also include dates of events in the months ahead, newcomers to the service, and thanks to those who are leaving. Volunteers can be encouraged to contribute to such a publication and this adds to the interest and the content of the newsletter. This newsletter could be published twice a year in-house at little cost if a computer and efficient printer are available.

Volunteer team leaders/coordinators

The larger organizations can benefit from a volunteer team leader/coordinator (TLC) system to help with the management of rotas and help with other events such as the orientation, induction, and training of volunteers. This system not only gives support to the VSM but also is another interesting way of supporting volunteers by providing a 'promotion' for those who are able and wish to become more involved in the management of the volunteer service. These areas are covered in more detail in Chapter 3.

This system has to be carefully organized and managed by the VSM with the selection of the TLCs being of utmost importance[2]. These volunteers, along with the volunteers, who have been selected to provide training for new volunteers will need an extra level of support from the VSM.

Regular meetings with the VSM should take place with all who help with such tasks. It is recommended that these meetings take place at least every 2 months. A social aspect can be added by having a meal together in the unit on the day of the meeting. This is a useful way of valuing those volunteers who take on the extra responsibility of helping the VSM in managing and training the volunteers.

Obvious as it sounds, all volunteers should be offered refreshments during their time on duty and if they spend more than 5 hours in a day, helping, then a meal also should be made available.

General support measures

It is important that the environment where the volunteers carry out their duties is adequately equipped. There should be available:

◆ Notice boards, with space dedicated to the volunteer services if it is a board for staff and volunteers, or a board in the volunteer office for information, the rosters for the different teams, and special notices.

◆ Appropriate equipment for the different duties done by volunteers, well maintained and simple to use and understand.

◆ Protective clothing should always be available with clear instructions for infection control procedures, hygiene, and any other protective measures required by the organization.

Much of this may be written in the Health and Safety handbook. Health and Safety responsibilities are covered in Chapter 8 on Legal Issues.

One of the most important and effective ways of supporting volunteers, as well as meeting them regularly, is to maintain an open door policy. Volunteers must know and understand that at any time volunteer office staff are available if a volunteer wants to see them. This contact is vital for teamwork and for giving confidence and trust in their support system.

Care must be taken not to abuse or take unfair advantage of the special commitment and flexibility that volunteers offer. Enthusiastic offers of help will soon wane if a volunteer is asked to do too much too often. This over-use of a volunteer can upset the balance of what is given and what a dedicated volunteer receives. Especially in palliative care, volunteers potentially may become over-involved with patients and families, contributing to the stressful time of loss for the volunteer when the patient dies.

Relationship with the VSM

The most important aspect of supporting volunteers during their time in the hospice is the relationship the volunteer has with the VSM and others who are connected with the voluntary service. The better the relationship, the more effectively the service will run. Individuals who manage volunteers need to have and to show interest in each and every volunteer. They must remember details of their volunteers' lives. The author would suggest that to store information about what has been called 'Grandchildren, Gran Canaria and Gall bladders' in one's memory can be very valuable. Such details about the families, the holidays, and the health of volunteers are not intrusive but can make a volunteer feel valued and important to the organization. When made to feel special, this helps them to appreciate their part in the larger team and, in turn, enhances their commitment and their sense of being wanted and appreciated.

Support when a volunteer is in difficulty

Volunteers who suffer crises in their lives need to be supported through them. This does not mean that the VSM needs a certificate in counselling, but should display a calm approach; have an empathetic listening ear, and be both available and approachable.

In the case of personal bereavement, it is necessary for volunteers to take time out until they feel ready to return. This need not be dealt with in a formal way. In the author's experience, volunteers who feel well supported are keen to come back sooner rather than later because of that support. They must feel comfortable to come back into the palliative care environment and it is the responsibility of the VSM to ensure that they do. The VSM will keep closely in touch with bereaved volunteers and until they wish to come back to their duties. At this point, the VSM should invite the volunteer to talk about how he/she feels about their loss and what support the volunteer feels may still be needed to help them to adjust. If there is doubt about the readiness to return, then volunteers should be urged to take more time; perhaps come in occasionally to help with duties, where they are not exposed to the nursing area of the unit. This can help the adjustment process. This support is always much appreciated and allows volunteers to come back to their own duties at the appropriate time, which varies from individual to individual. This consideration of the appropriateness of their wishes to return is a crucial process for the VSM. Very rarely a volunteer, having experienced a loss, will decide that the palliative care environment is no longer suitable for him/her and will withdraw. This wish must be respected.

In the event of illness, physical or mental, a volunteer, must be equally well supported. In palliative care, many volunteers first apply to join the voluntary service in middle age and may remain with the organization for many years. It is possible that not only may physical illnesses develop, which will affect their ability to work, but conditions, such as dementia, may occur. When this happens, sufferers may not be aware of the changes in their behaviour. The author has experienced four cases in 7 years in post and has some suggestions how to deal with this situation.

Dementia is progressive, and when it is first suspected, then staff and team leaders should be alerted and be made aware of difficulties that may arise. The time will come when the volunteer may need to be 'counselled out' of the organization. This can be hard to achieve without distress to everyone concerned. One method of dealing with this difficulty is by involving the family of the affected volunteer. A letter or telephone call or a meeting with the family will be necessary, giving reasons why their family member with dementia should not return to his/her volunteer duties. This contact should be promptly followed by a visit to the volunteer from the VSM with flowers or other suitable recognition, along with a 'thank you' letter. This usually works well and is appreciated by all.

Where there is no family support, the general practitioner (GP) may need to be involved. This needs the permission of the volunteer and requires to be approached very sensitively. Managing a volunteer with such a condition can be delicate but must be handled decisively to protect the volunteer and the organization from a difficult and possibly dangerous situation.

Any condition whether physical or mental, which causes the volunteer to be unable to carry out his/her duties effectively, must be addressed by the VSM. This may be done by inviting the volunteer to discuss his/her position in the volunteer team. It may be that permission needs to be sought to approach the GP of the volunteer in order to understand more about the situation. Sensitive handling of the situation can support the volunteer as he/she moves out of his/her present duty, but not necessarily out of the organization altogether. It may be possible to find tasks that are more suitable to the volunteer's capability. This solution benefits the organization, the voluntary service, and the volunteer.

In serious situations where theft, abuse of drugs or alcohol, or breaching the rules and procedures occur, these must be dismissed immediately. This is an obvious statement but crucial to observe to support others and the organization. This is especially important for the other volunteers who have duties alongside the offending volunteer. Such procedures must be outlined in the volunteer policy.

Support for volunteers when they leave the organization

In every palliative care unit where many volunteers are involved in many duties, there is ongoing turnover throughout the year. This is to be expected, acknowledged, and accepted as normal. It is useful for the VSM to offer an exit questionnaire to be completed by volunteers as they leave their duties. The benefits of this are that it:

◆ Allows the volunteer to be honest about their reasons for leaving.

◆ Gives an opportunity to state whether or not they felt supported during their time in the organization.

◆ Gathers feedback from the volunteer about the enjoyable and satisfactory experiences of their voluntary work.

◆ Gives the VSM an insight into criticisms of the service thus affording the opportunity to improve the service for all concerned.

Feedback of whatever nature is important when dealing with so many different individuals. The VSM and the staff concerned should always strive to improve the quality of the volunteer service to the organization.

If a volunteer retires because they are unhappy or feels badly dealt with, this must be taken very seriously. The VSM requires to investigate all aspects of the case to discover what has happened and to take steps to support the volunteer. There can be many reasons for such a situation, and the facts must be uncovered if the credibility of the voluntary service is not to be undermined. Moreover, generally, volunteers are very loyal and will leave an organization rather than make a stand against poor treatment or conditions. It is important for the reputation of the organization and its standing in the community that such problems are addressed. It could be of course that the volunteer management itself is the cause of stress to volunteers. This must be addressed and dealt with by the line manager of the VSM.

Everyone in the organization should recognize that volunteers, whether few or many, are a vital and effective relations group. They go out into the community with plenty to say about the organization and what they say has to be good. Supporting and valuing volunteers effectively can have considerable benefits for the unit in attracting people and funds to the organization. Volunteers taking their experiences into the community, report the quality of care, for patients, relatives, staff, and volunteers, for which palliative care is renowned.

Support for the VSM

This is a crucial issue for any volunteer service. Volunteers are more likely to be well managed if the VSM is also well managed and supported. Most palliative care units now recognize the importance of a dedicated volunteer manager who is paid, has a budget, is responsible for the volunteers in his/her care, and is accountable to the Chief Executive and or Board of Management for the service. Administrative support should be available as well as an office computer equipment with an effective database. The VSM should have regular support from and access to senior members of staff to discuss volunteer issues with them, ideally as a member of the senior management team. This ensures that volunteers are embedded in the strategy and policy of the hospice.

Conclusion

Volunteers come to help in palliative care units for many reasons. They bring a wide range of skills, experience, and personal qualities and come form all parts of the social spectrum.

Resources are needed to introduce, manage, and retain this valuable resource. The VSM must know his/her volunteers well and must encourage the staff of the organization to be sensitive, appreciative, and value the role played by volunteers.

There is no better feeling for a VSM than knowing a volunteer team is happy, supported, and appreciated by the staff involved and is giving dedication and commitment to the palliative care service.

This willing and generous gift of time to a hospice or palliative care unit by a large group of volunteers is one of the things that sets such places apart from other hospitals or care homes. Volunteers give invaluable assistance to the staff and help to create the special environment of peace and comfort appreciated by so many patients and relatives. To achieve optimal results, volunteers must themselves be fully and effectively supported.

References

1 McCurley, S. and Lynch, R. (1998). Appendix B. In *Essential Volunteer Management* (2nd edition), p. 211. London, Directory of Social Change.

2 Hamilton, G. (1997). Volunteering: Team leadership. *Hospice Bulletin*, April, p. 1. London, The Hospice Information Service, St. Christoper's Hospice.

Recommended reading

Adirondack, S. and Sinclair Taylor, J. (2001). *The Voluntary Sector Legal Handbook* (2nd edition). London, Directory of Social Change.

McCurley, S. and Lynch, R. (1998). *Essential Volunteer Management* (2nd edition). London, Directory of Social Change.

Chapter 8

Volunteering and legal issues

Mark Restall

Any information on the law runs the risk of being a put-off for potential readers. This chapter attempts to give an overview of the relevant areas of law in plain English. In doing so it may not meet the rigours of an academic article for legal professionals, but it is intended to give a working knowledge that will help voluntary services managers understand where they stand on day-to-day issues.

The legal position of volunteers has been a neglected area. Given the huge numbers of people who are involved as volunteers in the United Kingdom and the important role they play within society, this is a little strange; but then volunteer management as a whole has been a poor relation even within volunteer-involving organizations. On top of this, volunteers do not fall into a neat legal box. They are not employees, or customers, or service users. Some of the law involved is a little unclear as to how it applies to volunteers.

Yet the core issues are not beyond the reach of voluntary services managers, and it is important for hospices to have a decent understanding of their legal position with volunteers. Hospices are not a special case as such. Like any area where volunteers are involved they have their own context, but volunteer involvement in hospices is diverse, and I have not attempted to limit information to any stereotype of roles in this setting. Readers are cautioned that the author is not a lawyer in any shape or form. The information contained within is clearly not intended to be a substitute for professional legal advice.

Please note that this chapter refers to the law in England and Wales. This is does not significantly differ from the situation in Scotland or Northern Ireland, but readers are advised to check the situation with the respective national volunteering bodies.

Health and safety

Duty of care

Volunteers are not explicitly included within Health and Safety legislation in the same manner as employees. However, the responsibilities of hospices towards them are very high, and in terms of the law (let alone morality), there is no justification for taking any less care of volunteers.

Hospices have a 'duty of care' towards volunteers. The duty of care is a common law duty—this simply means that it comes through court decisions rather than an Act of Parliament. The duty of care is a duty to avoid carelessly causing harm or injury.

We all have this duty to the people around us, and volunteer-involving organizations owe this duty to their volunteers.

A more practical way of looking at the duty of care is that hospices should be taking all reasonable steps open to them to avoid volunteers coming to harm. It is worth noting the use of the term 'reasonable'. Volunteers do not have to be wrapped in cotton wool, and hospices do not have to follow the absurdities that popular culture ascribes to health and safety practice. Faced with making a decision as to whether a person or organization has been negligent, courts ask themselves the question 'could a reasonable person have foreseen this harm being caused'?

Health and safety at work etc Act 1974

In addition to the duty of care, under section 3 of the Health and Safety at Work Act, employers have a duty 'to ensure, so far as is reasonably practicable, that persons not in [their] employment who may be affected thereby are not thereby exposed to risks to their health or safety'[1].

Therefore, there is a duty under this key piece of Health and Safety legislation as well as the common law duty of care. In addition, there is also a duty to give people, who may be affected by an employer's work, any information relevant to their health and safety.

Risk assessments

Under the Management of Health and Safety at Work Regulations, 1999, employers must carry out risk assessments looking not only at the risks to employees, but also 'the risks to the health and safety of persons not in [their] employment arising out of or in connection with the conduct by him of his undertaking'. This, therefore, would include volunteers. Where the employer has five or more employees, the risk assessments must be written.

Written risk assessments on volunteer activities also help demonstrate that hospices are taking their duty of care seriously. The Health and Safety Executive suggests a five-step approach to risk assessment[2]:

1 Identify the hazards
2 Decide who might be harmed and how
3 Evaluate the risks and decide on precautions
4 Record your findings and implement them
5 Review your assessment and update if necessary

The 'compensation culture' and the Compensation Act 2006

In recent years, a general perception has arisen that we are living in a 'compensation culture'. Newspapers have splashed stories about ridiculous court cases, and their columnists regularly savage health-and-safety-based strictures on society. For voluntary and public sector organizations, this has led to concerns that they may be open to spurious claims made by service users or volunteers.

The actual evidence for a compensation culture is slim at best. In 2004 the government's Better Regulation Task Force published Better Routes to Redress. The foreword to this report stated:

> It is a commonly held perception that the United Kingdom is in the grip of a 'compensation culture'.... It is this perception that causes the real problem: the fear of litigation impacts on behaviour and imposes burdens on organizations trying to handle claims.
>
> The judicial process is very good at sorting the wheat from the chaff, but all claims must still be assessed in the early stages. Redress for a genuine claimant is hampered by the spurious claims arising from the perception of a compensation culture. The compensation culture is a myth; but the of this belief is very real.[3]

To help address this problem, the Compensation Act 2006 was introduced. It provides protection for organizations carrying out 'desirable activities'. In such cases courts considering claims for negligence or similar actions may take into account whether any steps that could have been taken to prevent the incident would have prevented the 'desirable activity' from going ahead in any meaningful way. Courts have in fact been pretty good at this, but the legislation was more aimed at reassurance than solving a genuine problem[4].

Other considerations

While not a legal requirement, volunteers should be explicitly included within the hospice's Health and Safety Policy. This both underlines commitment to the health and safety of volunteers and acts as a reminder to staff—especially those with senior responsibility for health and safety—that they must always include volunteers in any consideration of health and safety issues.

Health and safety issues should form part of induction and inform volunteer training—and indeed day-to-day supervision and more formal monitoring of the volunteer programme.

Criminal record checks

Many areas of the law around volunteering can seem unclear due to the lack of reference to volunteers in relevant legislation. With the law on criminal record checks and related vetting procedures, things are more clear-cut as volunteers are explicitly included. There has still been confusion for many volunteer-involving organizations as to when they should put volunteers through screening checks, but the advent of the Independent Safeguarding Authority (ISA) takes most of these tricky decisions out of the hands of volunteer managers.

Since 2002 the Criminal Records Bureau (CRB) has issued criminal record checks—disclosures—to employers and volunteer-involving organizations. Disclosures are only available where the following conditions are satisfied. Organizations seeking to obtain disclosures must follow the CRB code of practice, register with the CRB, or go through an approved 'umbrella body', and seek disclosures only for those roles they have an entitlement to check.

The Private and Voluntary Health Care (England) Regulations 2001 place a duty on hospices to carry out CRB checks on paid staff, but this does not extend to volunteers, as this duty applies only to those employed under the following definition:

> In these Regulations, references to employing a person include employing a person whether under a contract of service or a contract for services, and references to an employee or to a person being employed shall be construed accordingly.[5]

There are therefore two questions a voluntary services manager has to consider. Should we carry out a CRB disclosure? And are we allowed to do so?

The latter question is one that many volunteer-involving organizations fail to ask. Access to CRB disclosures is governed by whether or not the role that is being checked is included in the Rehabilitation of Offenders Act 1974 (Exceptions) Order 1975, which has been amended and updated many times over the years.

The purpose of the Exceptions Order was originally to set out those roles where applicants for certain positions could be asked to reveal their full criminal record history. Aside from more serious offences, most convictions are considered spent after a period of time. This means that they do not have to be disclosed to a future employer. The Exceptions Order listed the cases where organizations could ask about spent as well as unspent convictions.

This list of roles forms part of the CRB's Disclosure Information Pack for registered and umbrella bodies, and is available on their Web site (titled 'DIP 003 Disclosure Access Category Codes').

For children's hospices, anyone whose normal duties involve work within the hospice itself can be checked. This includes volunteers as well as paid staff. Such roles are one of eight 'regulated positions' defined under section 36 of the Criminal Justice and Court Services Act 2000: 'a position whose normal duties include work in ... a hospital which is exclusively or mainly for the reception and treatment of children'.

The definition of 'hospital' is taken from the National Health Service Act 1977— 'any institution for the reception and treatment of persons suffering from illness'.

The situation is different for adult hospices. A volunteer who regularly cares for, supervises, is involved in delivering training, or is in sole charge of a patient can be checked at enhanced level. Volunteers providing some kind of social-care service for patients can be checked at standard level.

What hospices must remember is that they may be involving volunteers in roles where a check is not permitted. An obvious area for many hospices would be charity shops. Seeking disclosures in such cases is a breach of the CRB's code of practice, not to mention the Police Act 1997, Rehabilitation of Offenders Act 1974 and Data Protection Act 1998.

Independent safeguarding authority and the vetting and barring scheme

At the time of writing this, the new scheme had not started. Therefore, some details had not yet been finalized, so readers are advised to refer to organizations such as Volunteering England and the ISA itself to ensure that they have the most up-to-date information.

The underlying legislation is unlikely to change much however, and it is this that I am concentrating on[6,7].

The Vetting and Barring Scheme (VBS) has been brought in following a recommendation of the Bichard Inquiry, set up after a high-profile murder case. The Safeguarding Vulnerable Groups Act 2006 has laid down the foundations and framework for this new screening regime and its accountable body, the ISA.

The 2006 Act defined two categories of roles associated with work involving children or vulnerable adults: 'regulated' and 'controlled' activities.

Regulated activities are specific roles when working with children or vulnerable adults either 'frequently', 'intensively', or 'overnight'. Frequently means at least once a month, intensively three or more times in any one month. These roles include: teaching, training, care, supervision, advice, treatment, and transportation, as well as work in specific settings, such as care homes and schools. These may be added to before (or after) the VBS starts operating.

Controlled activities are support roles in specific settings. They currently include:

◆ Frequent or intensive support work in general health settings, the NHS, and further education—e.g. cleaners, caretakers, catering staff, and receptionists.

◆ Individuals working for specified organizations (e.g. a local authority) who have frequent access to sensitive records about children and vulnerable adults.

◆ Support work in adult social-care settings. At present, according to my understanding, this relates to care homes and community care arranged by local authorities, rather than any organization that may work with vulnerable adults.

The initial vetting comes through registration with the scheme. Registration is carried out via the CRB, through a registered or umbrella body. This process involves an enhanced disclosure. If anything comes up through this check, the ISA will decide whether or not this information justifies barring the individual from working with children or vulnerable adults.

For some convictions there will be an automatic bar. In other cases, the ISA will allow the individual to make representation to them before the barring decision. Once a person is registered with the VBS, the CRB part of the process is bypassed—organizations can check their status directly online through the ISA. Organizations with regulated or controlled activities must report volunteers to the ISA where when they have dismissed an individual, or an individual resigns, because they harmed, or may harm, a child or vulnerable adult.

Hospices must decide whether they are satisfied with using the VBS system on its own. The CRB will still provide disclosures to organizations wanting to see a person's full criminal record history. It is too early to tell what common or accepted practice will be. Organizations such as Help the Hospices may be a source of guidance.

Equal opportunities and other employment protections

Employees are protected from discrimination on the grounds of race, gender, disability, sexual orientation, religion or belief, and age. None of this legislation extends this protection to volunteers. Most are also protected from unfair dismissal and have access to other rights such as maternity leave. Again, this legislation does not include volunteers—there is in law no such thing as an unfair dismissal of a volunteer.

The reason for this is that the relevant legislation does not provide the blanket protection from discrimination in all circumstances. The anti-discrimination legislation typically refers to discrimination in two settings—employment and (apart from the grounds of age) access to goods and services. Volunteering is not included in the definitions of employment used by such legislation. See the Section 'When is a volunteer not a volunteer?' for more information on this.

What this means for voluntary services managers is that there is therefore a moral rather than legal responsibility on their part to ensure that volunteers are treated fairly. Volunteers should be included within equal opportunities/diversity policies, and good practice followed in recruitment and the support and supervision of volunteers. As hospices may be liable for the actions of their volunteers if an employee or patient experiences discrimination of some form, it is important that volunteers are given a full understanding of the behaviour expected of them in this regard.

There are some possibilities for action from volunteers who feel that they have been discriminated against or poorly treated. The possibility has been raised that volunteers could claim that the treatment they experienced could be seen as discrimination in terms of access to a service. This would mean arguing that involving volunteers amounted to providing a service for them. This has never been tested and remains an unlikely route for redress.

Where a volunteer has suffered mental or emotional harm as a result of their time spent volunteering there may be the chance to argue that their organization has failed its health and safety duties. I know of no such case being brought however.

Volunteers who have suffered bullying or similar harassment at work may be able to use the Protection from Harassment Act 1997. Although this act was initially brought in to prevent stalking, it has been successfully used by an employee to find their employer 'vicariously liable' for their harassment from another member of staff[8]. As this legislation is not based on any definitions of employment, there is in theory no reason why a volunteer could not make use of it.

Expenses

Reimbursement of volunteer expenses is considered to be good practice. It ensures that volunteering is open to all, regardless of income. Care should be taken to reimburse volunteers for their actual costs—collecting receipts or other evidence where possible.

Flat rate expenses—that is, giving a fixed sum such as £5 per day—should be avoided. Money over and above out-of-pocket expenses will be treated as income by HM Revenue and Customs (HMRC) and Jobcentre Plus, and may change the relationship with the volunteer, giving them employment status[9].

Vehicle costs may be reimbursed up to the approved mileage rate set by HMRC—at the time of writing this was 40 p per mile for cars, but this figure is overdue for reassessment. The figure is set to allow employees (and in this case volunteers) to be reimbursed for their travel without tax implications[10].

Benefits claimants

The rules for benefits claimants who wish to volunteer are fairly straightforward, and should not present a barrier. However, problems can arise when volunteers come up against poorly informed benefits advisers, so it is important for voluntary services managers to keep up to date on this issue[11].

There are some areas of confusion that may affect claimants on any benefit. It is commonly held (even by benefits advisers) that there is a 16 hour limit on volunteering whilst in receipt of benefits. This is not true. Most information produced on volunteering by Jobcentre Plus will now say something along these lines '... you can volunteer as many hours as you like while you are on benefits as long as you still meet the terms for getting them'[11].

It may still be prudent for claimants to avoid volunteering full time—benefits advisers may see this as evidence that they are not looking for work [if they are on Jobseeker's Allowance(JSA)] or are actually fit for work (if on Incapacity Benefit or the 'Support Group' element of Employment and Support Allowance).

The only genuine hour limit, however, is for people in receipt of Carer's Allowance—their volunteering must not interfere with the 35 hours of caring they must provide each week[11].

One other issue that is rarer but does occasionally arise is a misunderstanding over what kind of organizations a claimant is allowed to volunteer for. Hospices that are part of an NHS trust may face this, as the confusion arises under a belief that claimants can only volunteer for a charity—sometimes this is refined to 'registered charity'. This appears to arise from the use of two complementary definitions in some legislation and Jobcentre Plus internal guidance:

> 'volunteer' means a person who is engaged in voluntary work with a charity or voluntary organization, or who is engaged in voluntary work otherwise than for a close relative, where the only payment received by him or due to be paid to him by virtue of being so engaged in respect of any expenses reasonably incurred by him in connection with that work[12]

Note that there are two definitions—the latter is broader and would include public sector bodies as well as the voluntary sector. In fact, elsewhere the former definition would include the statutory sector as well:

> 'voluntary work' means work for an organization the activities of which are carried on otherwise than for profit, or work other than for a member of the claimant's family ...[13]

Jobseekers Allowance claimants must remain available for and actively seeking work. There is a concession for volunteers over availability. Rather than having to be available to start work or attend an interview 'immediately' they have 48 hours notice to attend an interview and a week's notice to start a job. To demonstrate that they are actively seeking work claimants must take steps to look for work each week. As long as they are still doing so, volunteering should not affect their JSA claim.

Volunteers in receipt of Incapacity Benefit or its replacement, Employment and Support Allowance, are fully entitled to volunteer without their claim being affected—at least according to the relevant regulations. It is not unheard of for claimants to face problems from Jobcentre staff unaware of the rules on volunteering.

The legislation describes volunteering as 'exempt work' in regulation 45 (6) of the Employment and Support Allowance Regulations 2008 and regulation 17 (1)(b) of the The Social Security (Incapacity for Work) (General) Regulations 1995.

The situation is similar for all other benefits—as long as the individual continues to meet the requirements of their benefit, volunteering should not affect their claim in any way[11]. Note that claimants should inform the Jobcentre that they are volunteering. It is not the place or responsibility of a hospice voluntary services manager to ensure that they have done so, but they should be made aware of this, as complications could arise for the individual if the Jobcentre found out at a later date.

When is a volunteer not a volunteer?

This subtitle is no joke. There have been a handful of cases where an employment tribunal has decided that a particular volunteer or volunteers were employed in the eyes of the law, and therefore entitled to some or all employment rights. There are also anecdotal accounts of minimum wage inspectors warning organizations that their volunteers were workers under the National Minimum Wage Act.

The reason that this can occur is due to the way employment is defined in law. Employment is a legal relationship, based on there being a contract in place between the employer and employee.

We tend to think of contracts as being specific documents, perhaps drafted by lawyers and signed by both parties. While it is true that for important matters we do have written 'contracts', it's more accurate to think of these documents as descriptions of the contract. A contract is a relationship. It can arise without either party necessarily realizing that this has happened.

For a contract to be in place, there has to be 'consideration' and 'intent'. Consideration means the exchange of something of value. This is not limited to money, although that is its typical form. Intent refers to an intention to enter a binding relationship. This does not mean that the parties have to have expressed this—intent can be inferred from the actual circumstances of the relationship if there are clear obligations involved.

There are in effect two tiers of employment described by legislation. There is a broader definition of employment used by the employment provisions of the anti-discrimination legislation, the National Minimum Wage Act 1999, and the Working Time Regulations 1998. This is a contract to personally provide services. Some people may be employed under this definition, yet not have full employment rights. The term 'worker' is often used to describe this category.

The Employment Rights Act 1996 and related legislation use a narrower definition of employment – a 'contract of service'. It is much harder to define this form of contract, arising as it does from common law. I apologize in advance to legal professionals for this simplification, but two key elements to be considered (particularly around volunteering) are 'control' and 'mutuality of obligation'. Control refers to the amount of control the employer has over the 'employee'. Is the organization directing the how, when, and where of the work? 'Mutuality of obligation' refers to a mutual obligation to provide and carry out work.

Employees under this definition have access to protection from unfair dismissal, maternity entitlements, sick pay—the full range of employment rights.

There have only been a handful of cases involving volunteers. Space precludes going into detail on earlier cases[15], but the most important recent case offers a good overview of the current position. *South East Sheffield Citizen's Advice Bureau v Grayson [2004] IRLR 353* was an Employment Appeal Tribunal (EAT) case looking at a prior tribunal case that found the Bureau's volunteers could be regarded as employed under the Disability Discrimination Act.

In summary, the tribunal's decision was reached on the basis that:

'... there was an intention that work would be done by the advisers in return for the payment of expenses incurred and the provision of training, the opportunity to gain experience and the acceptance of legal liability on the part of the Bureau for any errors which they may commit in the course of the work done.'[16]

The tribunal also pointed to the existence of disciplinary and grievance procedures, equal opportunities and health and safety policies, and provision for supervision as being consistent with employment.

The Appeal Tribunal took a different view. Perhaps the key to its judgement can be seen in the way it highlighted a phrase within the CAB's Volunteer Agreement, that it was there '... to clarify the reasonable expectations of both the volunteer and the Bureau'.

As an example of a 'reasonable expectation' the Tribunal looked at the minimum time commitment of 6 hours of voluntary work per week that the CAB expressed. As this was described as a 'usual minimum commitment', and that there were no sanctions on those who, for whatever reason, could not meet that commitment at some point, the Tribunal looked on this as an expectation rather than a binding obligation. In fact, it noted that the Bureau relied on volunteers and that, therefore, it was not unreasonable for it to set out such guidelines.

The original tribunal's view of the consideration element, which it saw in the relationship was similarly treated. The training was felt to be relevant to the role the volunteers carried out, and not felt to be a reciprocal 'perk' in return for the work the volunteers provided. The EAT also stated that it 'cannot understand' the view of experience gained as a form of consideration.

On expenses, the EAT noted that the expenses payments made by the Bureau were the reimbursement of actual expenses, going so far as to say:

It would, in our view, be very surprising if unpaid volunteers were expected to bear their expenses incurred in the course of their work for the Bureau, and we do not regard this feature of the Agreement as providing support for the contention that in truth the Agreement was one of service or for the personal provision of services.[16]

This EAT case has proved fairly robust, with at least two subsequent cases involving volunteers basing their judgement upon it. However, this does not mean that no volunteers in the future will be able to prove that they have employment status.

Hospices, therefore, need to ensure that volunteers are reimbursed for out-of-pocket expenses only, and that they are not receiving other appreciable perks. Training should be related to the work volunteers are carrying out, and there should not be qualifying time periods before or after it is provided. The relationship itself should be described in terms of expectation rather than obligation. Organizations such as Volunteering England can provide examples of Volunteer Agreements and other documents written in such language.

Further information

Volunteering England information service www.volunteering.org.uk
National Volunteering Infrastructure Body
Volunteers and the Law Mark Restall
Free in-depth publication available from Volunteering England
The Russell-Cooke Voluntary Sector Legal Handbook (3rd edition) Ed. Sandy Adirondack
Forthcoming at the time of writing, available from Directory of Social Change.

References

1 *Health and Safety at Work etc Act 1974.*
2 Health and Safety Executive. (2006). *Five Steps to Risk Assessment.* London, HSE.
3 Better Regulation Task Force. (2004). *Better Routes to Redress.* London, BTRF.
4 *Compensation Act 2006.*
5 *The Private and Voluntary Health Care (England) Regulations* 2001, s2 (3).
6 *Safeguarding Vulnerable Groups Act 2006.*
7 Independent Safeguarding Authority Web site: www.isa-gov.org.uk, last accessed in October 2008.
8 *Majrowski v St Guy's and St Thomas' NHS Trust [2006] UKHL 34.*
9 Volunteering England. (2008). *Volunteer Expenses Information Sheet.* London, VE.
10 HMRC Web site: http://www.hmrc.gov.uk/mileage/volunteer-drivers.htm, last accessed in October 2008.
11 Volunteering England. (2008). *Volunteering and State Benefits Information Sheet.* London, VE.
12 Jobcentre Plus. (2008). *Volunteering while Receiving Benefits.* London, Jobcentre Plus.
13 *The Social Security (Incapacity for Work) (General) Regulations 1995.*
14 *The Jobseeker's Allowance Regulations 1996.*
15 Restall, M. (2005). *Volunteers and the Law.* London, Volunteering England.
16 *South East Sheffield Citizen's Advice Bureau v Grayson [2004] IRLR 353* available at http://www.employmentappeals.gov.uk/Public/Upload/UKEAT2830317112003.doc, last accessed October 2008.

Chapter 9

Professionals working as volunteers

Silke Lean and Patricia McDermott

Very little has been published about the issues surrounding professionals who wish to contribute their professional skills as volunteers in a hospice/palliative care service—their selection, training, supervision, accountability, and the many planning issues that inevitably arise. It is important to avoid wasting the time of volunteers, as there is nothing as a rule that they hate more, and this is even truer of professional volunteers. But this is exactly what happens if there has been insufficient planning and vision to define and prepare for the work to be done.

This chapter will examine some of the factors that affect the integration of professional volunteers in a palliative care unit.

Why have professional volunteers?

Volunteering appears to be going through some changes related to the style in which people choose to participate. We are moving towards a system in which there are two distinct types of volunteers: (1) the long-term volunteer, who lives locally and has been trained in-house to provide a specific support task, and (2) the specialist volunteer bringing externally acquired expertise in to a hospice.

Specialist volunteering is gaining a higher profile with more people becoming aware of the option of donating not just their time, but a specific skill. This coincides with recent economic trends, which have heightened the commitment of palliative care units to make volunteering more effective.

As the definition and use of the word 'volunteer' changes, let us start by defining what we mean when we talk about professional volunteers in palliative care. This is a person that donates his/her specialist skills and time for a charitable purpose, mostly, although not exclusively to enhance the quality of physical care that is provided for patients.

The main reason why professional volunteers are such an asset in palliative care is because they donate their time and skills cost-free. They are obviously saving resources but crucially help a palliative care unit to provide additional skills and services that could not be funded out of the core budget.

Involving volunteers that are highly skilled, often in an area that is not economically viable to attract funding, gives unique opportunities to extend the quality and range of care that can be offered to patients and relatives.

In what way are volunteers donating a professional skill different?

All the management principles that work effectively with volunteers apply to professional volunteers as well, but some of the common problems with volunteer involvement are thrown into sharper focus with professional placements.

These volunteers are likely to have a high expectation of being managed well, because they compare how their skill is valued in the marketplace. They are often highly skilled and are motivated to improve their skills in a specialist setting and have a good understanding of the value of their skill to the voluntary sector. This, in turn, leads to expectations to have an equal relationship with paid professional staff and have their opinions heard and acted on. They are confident in their approach and expect to have a certain amount of influence in the organizational decision-making process.

There is a growing trend to professionalize volunteer involvement and management. There are now different expectations from the senior management team in a palliative care unit about volunteer involvement, which coincide with changes in the economic climate. Palliative care units are constantly undergoing financial reviews, which has led to re-evaluating the workings of the multidisciplinary team. Professional volunteers as part of the team now not only complement but may also extend core services.

We are also more inclined to follow the examples of some of the large-scale volunteer programmes found in the United States of America. There is a much greater emphasis on realizing the cost–benefit relationship of volunteering and measuring the value of donated time to a charity, which is then offset against project funding.

What kind of professional volunteer can be utilized?

There is potentially an endless list of people than can be involved and the variety of professionals on the team will be a combination of the vision of potential by the unit, of who applies, who is recruited, and who is successfully integrated and stays. Some examples, but by no means an exclusive list, are: health-care workers, counsellors, physiotherapists, interpreters, receptionists, art and music therapists, hairdressers, beauticians. There is another, in most cases smaller, group of professional volunteers who work in non-patient care roles: for example, accountants, secretaries, and librarians.

For some professionals, the motivation to donate their skills is similar to any volunteers. But for others it gives the opportunity to gain new experiences, develop, update their skills, and utilize them in a different context.

Recent trends suggest that there is a decline in the number of traditional 'not professionally educated and trained' female middle-class volunteers who used to be the mainstay of additional help in a palliative care unit. Women are more likely to be involved in direct patient care than are men. Some of the changes in our society mean that more well-educated women now often have a professional career and balance this with family life. This means that a larger group of women with professional skills may now be available, wishing to donate time to a charity in their professional capacity.

Complementary therapy is one of the areas were where professional volunteer services are increasing. Whilst this service has enhanced care and is clearly popular with patients, it has led to the need to promote safe good practice in their clinical management.

Palliative care units are also seeing an increase in employee volunteering and second-ments. Practice varies, but a typical employee volunteer will donate his/her professional skill for a few hours a month where it is needed, perhaps research a specific project or sit on a committee. Secondments are short- to medium-term placements, often to assist in aspects of strategic planning and management.

Another demographic trend points to an increasingly older population, some of whom may retire early. This means not only will there be a greater need for services for older people, but crucially that there will be a larger pool of active volunteers to draw on. These retired professionals can be recruited to provide a rich source of expertise and skills.

Whatever the ultimate aims are for professional volunteer involvement, it is good management practice to start small. It makes sense to pilot new procedures and deal with problems that will only surface once a new placement has been introduced.

Case study: Introducing a new therapy

Katie is a qualified Reiki practitioner who has worked with patients for the last 10 years. She has her own thriving private practice and works from home, but she is keen to donate some of her time and skills to cancer patients. She is affiliated to the World Federation of Healing, which provides her with access to specialist insurance and support.

The concept of healing in working with patients who are suffering from life-threatening conditions or terminally ill patients has always been controversial, with the unspoken assumption that it raises false hopes of a cure. But as awareness of complementary therapies has become greater in the general population, the idea does get mentioned both by patients and potential volunteers who offer to provide this service. In this circumstance, the word 'healing' takes on a somewhat different meaning, emphasizing a return to greater wholeness, relaxation, and well-being. After the interview and verification of Katie's qualifications, references, and experience, Reiki as a specialty was discussed with the multidisciplinary team. As the demand for this therapy was patient-led, a trial placement was agreed.

Utilizing Katie's professional skills gave patients access to another therapy, which would not have been funded by a palliative care provider. Through Katie's teaching and feedback from patients, staff were able to understand more about Reiki and its value for patients. The staff had to learn to manage a professional volunteer and reassess how they work as a team.

Case study: Introducing a new therapy *(continued)*

Issues arose about access to patient information, referral forms, job title, working space, and involvement in multidisciplinary meetings. All of these issues had to be resolved as a team and many are ongoing.

Reiki remains a popular therapy in the unit but is considered to be a controversial concept by many professionals.

This is an example of how a professional volunteer can be integrated into a team to offer a service that is not considered to be mainstream but one that more and more patients in a palliative care setting demand.

The application process

The most important step in deciding whether a professional volunteer will fit the team is by meeting face to face. This should precede written documentation and a formal interview. From a visit you can start to see an individual's personality and form an opinion whether someone will integrate into an existing team. It will be possible to pick up on what is motivating the potential applicant and what they expect from the palliative care unit. It may be that after an informal visit the volunteer decides not to apply, perhaps the unit does not meet his/her needs. If this is the case, then the visit has been of value as it has saved you and them a great deal of time. It is important that the applicants at this stage read the volunteer policy, which should detail their responsibilities. If they are not happy with the policy, then there is little point in continuing with the application process.

Recruiting professional volunteers involves devising an appropriate, comprehensive application form, which supplies details a palliative care unit must have before accepting a professional volunteer.

It is crucial to know:

◆ Qualifications

◆ Professional background

◆ Colleges/Schools

◆ Insurance

◆ Their motivations and expectations

Ask about colleges, as some have a better reputation than others do and get information on the content of courses such as:

◆ How long is the course?

◆ Does it involve client contact?

◆ What is required before enrolment?

◆ What qualification do people graduate with?

The references taken up should be from someone who can comment on the professional's practice. If the applicant is a therapist then, ideally, one of the references should be from a former tutor. This information gives a good idea of how the professional works and whether his/her style of working will fit the unit. It is important to check your organization's insurance policy as to whether specialist volunteer work is covered. If it is a volunteer complementary therapist, they are likely to be affiliated to a professional body and have the option to take out personal insurance which may cover them whilst volunteering. Copies of the insurance policy must be kept on the volunteer file and updated annually. It is worth remembering that an established team has its own dynamics. A new recruit with a different style of working, especially if they introduce a new treatment, can cause major upheaval. Ensure that the team understands what motivates a particular professional and assess whether the palliative care team can offer that experience. Specialist volunteers need support, supervision, and training. In many ways, this is no different to what all volunteers need. However, a professional qualification may need updating and this has a cost implication. These costs need to be considered before the volunteer is recruited. An application process does not only consist of a completed application form but should involve an interview that will not just request but more crucially receive information from the professional volunteer. A volunteer with a specialty in a particular area will be a valuable addition to the service that is provided but will make greater demands on staff's time and resources.

Relations between paid and unpaid staff

The working relationships between staff teams are without doubt the most important factor in determining the success of professional placements. There are a number of reasons why paid staff might feel threatened by professional volunteers or, in turn, volunteers may be resistant to work well with employees.

Sometimes, paid staff assume that if someone works without payment he/she cannot be very good at what he/she does, while assuming that another paid member of the team is competent unless it is proven otherwise. The 'I am only a volunteer' syndrome is unhelpful. Volunteers must have feedback that they are an essential and valued part of the team. This also means giving unpaid members of staff a title and name badge that reflects the job they do.

Volunteers should be invited by name to relevant team meetings. Their professional opinions should be listened to and they must be involved in planning decisions that affect their work. If volunteers are not involved in the planning and decision-making process and acquire a sense of ownership of their projects and patients, their motivation and pride of their achievements will diminish. Also, if there is lack of consistency in their management, different supervising staff working to different rules, this will mean that volunteers become confused, resentful, and powerless. This is especially true of volunteers that only work infrequent shifts.

If volunteers are highly trained in the skill they are donating, they can be perceived as a threat by inexperienced staff, with the implication that they might be difficult to manage. This can be avoided through effective two-way communication. As a member of the team, a professional volunteer can be an equal member of the team and can be an effective educator to other staff.

Any one who works or volunteers in health-care settings knows the importance of confidentiality. It is a curious assumption that unpaid professional staff cannot be trusted with confidential information, and are more likely to be indiscreet. This attitude will be extremely divisive, as professional volunteers are no more likely to discuss their work than any other staff. Signing an agreement, appropriate training, and generating a forum for discussions will go some way towards reducing concerns. All paid and unpaid staff should work in an environment in which they have access to the information they 'need to know' to do their job. There should be no distinction for volunteers.

Supervision

The effectiveness of any volunteer programme is dependent on the quality of supervision volunteers receive. To ensure that professional volunteers can work effectively, it is necessary to concentrate on building relationships that respect and recognize the competency and professionalism of all staff in the multidisciplinary team. Who is the best line manager to evaluate a specialty? It may take some serious consideration to find the most appropriate person to comment on another's clinical or non-clinical work. Careful thought should be given to the whole idea of supervision. If it cannot be provided internally, there will be a cost implication.

Accountability

In the case of volunteers trained and working as health-care professionals (doctor, nurse, physiotherapist, etc.), they should logically be accountable to their clinical line manager. The doctor is accountable to the senior doctor, the nurse to the senior nurse, and so on. What is not so obvious and therefore requires careful thought and planning before the volunteer starts work, is to whom a complementary therapist is accountable, a librarian, a computer specialist, a hairdresser, or beautician. Whatever is decided must be explained to the volunteers before they start their work.

Grievances and discipline

Professional volunteers should be treated in a similar way to paid staff when it comes to grievances or disciplinary issues. It is important to have a role description for each placement, which defines expectations of the standard and quality of the work expected. If there is a suggestion that a professional volunteer is not performing or adhering to policies or procedures, the organization's disciplinary procedure appropriate to volunteers should be put into action. The fact that a professional works unpaid may lead supervising staff to be more lenient in dealing with performance issues, which should not be the case. This also applies to reviews or appraisals. Any professional will expect constructive feedback on their work. Consideration must be given, however, to the issues outlined in Chapter 8, in ensuring that language and structure of procedures that relate to volunteers in any capacity, do not indicate the existence of a contract of employment.

Case study: Paid and volunteer nurses working in the same team

Norman is a registered nurse who has recently retired early due to a minor medical problem. He loves being with patients and enjoyed a successful career in a large teaching hospital. When he approached his local palliative care unit he found that using volunteer nurses had not been considered. He was recruited as a general volunteer on the wards, talking to patients, making tea and coffee, and doing various other volunteer duties. It soon became obvious that Norman had a lot more to offer and he expanded his role slowly. He helped to make beds, wash and shave patients, and assisted the nurses, as they required. The extra help was generally welcomed, but some staff were concerned that his extended role was not part, and should not be part, of what volunteers should do. Some nurses were also concerned about how using unpaid staff might affect their jobs. As in many hospices, the unit was undergoing changes and cutbacks had been made. Serious issues were raised like insurance cover, access to confidential notes, and meetings. The staff were concerned for Norman's safety and highlighted potential problem areas including manual handling, risk assessment, and infection control.

Further discussions with staff generated greater insight into their views on working with professional volunteers. It was made clear that volunteer nurses would always be additional to accepted staffing levels, and would be able to take some pressure off the rest of the team, but would never substitute for paid staff. The staff, in this case, were not happy for Norman to attend their team meetings to discuss, plan, and evaluate care and they felt he was not, therefore, fully aware of issues surrounding patient needs.

The role of the volunteer in a nursing capacity that is an equal member of the nursing teams is one that this unit is not ready for. It would not be helpful to continue to advocate this type of nursing placement until the staff and management are fully supportive and keen to make it work. A compromise was reached where Norman can make good use of his experience and skills without being subjected to the same pressures as the nursing staff.

Funding and facilities

When involving volunteers it is important to examine carefully the implications of having new members on the team. This is especially true when recruiting professional staff. They will expect the appropriate facilities and funding for the work they are proposing to do. Important considerations are access to desks and computers, availability of treatment rooms for therapists, lockers and changing rooms, uniforms, aprons, or other protective clothing. Also, the cost of paying for equipment can be very high, depending on the skill being offered. If you are planning to recruit a hairdresser, you might well find they expect some of the equipment they are accustomed to in their working life outside the organization. Think about height-adjustable chairs, sinks, large mirrors, and pleasant surroundings. Consider whether the patients pay a contribution to this, often very popular service or whether it will be offered without charge.

Another often forgotten cost is the option to contribute to the insurance cover for therapists, especially if they are newly qualified and do not have their own practice. By far the largest underestimated resource implication is the hidden cost of the management, support, and supervision of professional volunteers. To make the service work, volunteers need to have induction, on-the-job training, briefing and debriefing, and time for support sessions. Multiply this by the number of volunteers and then add the turnover. Further allow for the fact that they do about one shift per week and hence have different communication and update needs than full-time staff. You arrive at a substantial number of hours.

Is volunteer management included in paid staff job descriptions and, if not, will the staff find the time to look after the professional volunteers allocated to their department? Ward managers may feel that volunteers drain staff time from their real work. Specialist volunteers do need access to a supervisor. If a member of permanent staff finds that their manager is busy, the question can probably wait a while. But a volunteer may only be in the unit once a week. In that situation, a huge amount of time and, by implication, money is wasted if the volunteer cannot get on with their designated work.

Writing a policy about involving professional volunteers

Any written policy is an essential framework for good practice. When writing a policy collectively you gain a consensus of opinion, thus facilitating an optimal volunteer environment, which ensures that paid and unpaid staff work together with clear goals and expectations.

The starting point for working with professional volunteers is in some ways no different than working with volunteers who have no specialist skills or training. Identifying where help is required, defining what that help is, highlighting the skills required, and evaluating the success of the project or placement remains crucial to any successful volunteer initiative. However, when working with professional volunteers, there are a number of other key factors that need to be given careful consideration. These include:

- Volunteer expectations of volunteering.
- Staff ideas and reservations about working with an unpaid professional.
- Boundaries and frameworks within which the volunteer operates.
- Confidentiality and clinical information sharing. It is hard to look at these issues when the volunteer is already working. It is far better practice to define key responsibilities before the volunteer commences his/her placement. The easiest way to do that is to write a policy.

Who should write the policy and who is it for?

It is best to have a group of people involved in a project like this. This way you will have a comprehensive, objective document. It is important to have a chairperson and someone to take detailed minutes. Policies should be working documents and are therefore subject to regular review by the policy writers. Depending on the size of the organization, a number of senior members of staff should be included to discuss strategic issues and certainly some representatives from the professions in question. The policy should be written to define key responsibilities, so that the paid and unpaid staff working together knows exactly what is expected of them.

What will be the content of the policy?

Included in the policy document should be the following:

◆ The title.

◆ The policy statement defining what we aim to achieve.

◆ The purpose.

◆ Definitions of the professions in question.

◆ The referral system.

◆ Patient consent and confidentiality.

◆ The responsibility of the volunteer, paid staff, and line manager.

◆ Criteria for accepting a volunteer in a professional capacity, including qualifications and experience required.

Consider the issue that although professionals may want to help, they will probably also want to expand their own paid private work. Is it acceptable to use the palliative care unit to make new contacts? What of the patient who is being discharged home but who wants to continue receiving the volunteer's aroma-therapy or reflexology? The whole issue of the professional volunteer's boundary needs to be discussed and addressed before placement starts.

Conclusion

This chapter has highlighted some of the issues that need to be considered when using volunteers in palliative care, working in a professional capacity. It presents the challenge to utilize donated time and skills to the maximum, because volunteers cannot fully and successfully contribute to a hospice unless they are recognized and planned for by the management and staff. This points to certain dilemmas and each unit needs to weigh up the costs and benefits involved and decide how they would cope. Does the palliative care unit have the staff resources and commitments to supervise professional volunteers? These are key issues.

> **Key issues: Considerations when planning volunteer placements**
>
> ◆ Have a role description in place for the placements you wish to recruit for.
> ◆ Identify line management responsibilities for professional roles.
> ◆ Ensure appropriate funding and facilities.
> ◆ Consider support and supervision needs.
> ◆ Write a policy.
> ◆ Training on confidentiality.
> ◆ Incorporate volunteer management issues in staff training.

Volunteering trends point to the fact that volunteering is becoming more professional, and expectations and standards are becoming more defined. The role of the Voluntary Services Manager (VSM) has been extended to plan ahead, evaluate, and anticipate potential concerns. This is a change from the traditional role of direct volunteer supervision. Teaching staff about the management of professional volunteers has become a major aspect of the VSM's role.

A final thought. People are an organization's greatest asset and professional volunteers can potentially bring great benefits to service provision. The question is not whether volunteers can fill gaps in the budget, but whether a palliative care unit is truly prepared to utilize volunteers in teamwork with paid staff. The notion that professional volunteers offer a 'free service' remains one of the greatest challenges in planning for volunteer involvement.

Chapter 10

Ethical issues for VSMs in hospice care

Steve McCurley and Ros Scott

Introduction

We often focus on volunteer involvement as a system for providing services to patients, a focus that is simple to do in hospices where the needs of the patient are often straight-forward and obvious. Voluntary Services Managers (VSMs) in hospices then address their own attention to the classic tasks of volunteer management: designing roles for volunteers, recruiting, induction and training, and providing a supervisory and support system.

Within all these tasks, however, lurk a number of less obvious and much more subtle issues, many of which require decisions based on ethics and values-based considerations. These decisions are made not only by the VSMs but also by the other parties involved in the process of providing care—hospice staff, patients and family members, and volunteers themselves.

In this chapter, we will examine some examples of ethical issues affecting the involvement of volunteers in hospices and suggest some practical means though which VSMs can assist both themselves and others as they work their way through decisions about the ethics and boundaries of good conduct.

Ethics and volunteer involvement

Ethics is the process by which values and principles are transformed into action. Ethical values provide the decision maker with a means of determining what is right versus what is wrong. The field of volunteer management—like most professional fields—has produced a variety of its own codes of ethical behaviour. In the United States, the Association for Volunteer Administration[1] suggested the following core ethical values for those who mobilize, direct, and motivate volunteers:

1 Citizenship and philanthropy

2 Respect

3 Responsibility

4 Compassion and generosity

5 Justice and fairness

6 Trustworthiness

In Canada, the British Columbia Hospice Palliative Care Association[2] enunciated a standard for ethical behaviour of volunteers in hospice programmes:

> Standard One: Competence
> C. Ethics: You are confident that you are carrying out your responsibilities within the ethical guidelines of your organization and the setting in which you volunteer. Volunteers are oriented to and understand all ethical guidelines related to hospice palliative care including:
> 1 Confidentiality and privacy
> 2 Boundaries to the relationship between volunteer and patient/family
> 3 Ethical guidelines specific to each of the settings in which they volunteer.

Neither of these sets of ethical principles is apt to provoke much argument—each provides a standard of action that seems admirable and appropriate.

As in many philosophical determinations, however, the difficulty lies not in stating ethical principles, but in practically applying them.

Ethical issues and conflicts in managing volunteers

Difficulties can arise in making ethical decisions in a variety of ways:

- Differing ethical values are held by various parties involved in the situation.
- Conflicts exist between the ethical values held by an individual.
- Grey areas of interpretation exist within ethical principles.

We will briefly examine some examples of these difficulties, focusing first on conflicts for the volunteer programme and its operation and, secondly, for the individual volunteer.

Conflicts for the volunteer programme

As VSMs go about their operation of the volunteer programme they face a number of ethical issues. Some of these conflicts are minor, and may affect only the volunteer manager. Merrill[3], for example, tells the following story:

> A long-time volunteer asked me if she could use my name for an employment reference. She has been with us for a long time and I know her well as a friend. She's a good person and a dependable volunteer. But, I am very uncomfortable about giving a job reference. I do not feel she has the skills or ability to tackle the job she is seeking. I would personally never hire her for that job. That's not to say she wouldn't be great in a lot of other things. But this position is not where her strengths lie. So what do I do?

Some of the ethical conflicts, however, can pose quite substantial issues for the VSM. These include:

1 Determination of appropriate roles for volunteers:

Volunteer management has always held that volunteers are a means of supplementing not supplanting paid staff roles. This ethical principle—the protection of the right of individuals to fair employment—is supported both by VSMs and by volunteers. In practice, however, this is a difficult issue, especially in very small charitable organizations, where changes in funding may often necessitate alterations in how and by whom work is done. Further complicating this issue is the interest of current and prospective patients of hospices in receiving service—if funding cuts results in staff redundancy is it then right or wrong to utilize volunteers to provide services to patients who would otherwise not receive assistance?

Related to this issue is the question of appropriate behaviour by volunteers during industrial actions or work stoppages—should the VSM engage volunteers in providing service during such actions or should the volunteers cease work as well?

2 Determination of how volunteers will be managed:

One challenge for new hospice organizations is the question of whether volunteer involvement has been considered and planned rather that developing organically. Have volunteers been given the same consideration in terms of management and support as paid staff? Who will manage the volunteers: will this be added to an already existing busy role or will a dedicated person with volunteer management experience be appointed? Availability of funding may be the determining factor in how volunteers will be managed. However, considering the challenging environment and the sensitivity of volunteer roles, one key ethical consideration for hospices is how they ensure their commitment to volunteers by ensuring safe, effective, and knowledgeable management.

3 Matching of volunteers and patients:

Volunteer/patient relationships are a delicate act of matching for compatibility. Grey areas exist, however, in determining exactly what factors are appropriate in making this match and what factors ought not to be allowed. Suppose, for example, that a particular patient (or volunteer, since this could come from either party) expresses a strong preference that their volunteer be of a particular ethnic or cultural grouping (or not be from a particular group). Is adhering to this preference simply good management—allowing for greater compatibility, better communication, and understanding—or would it be abetting a form of discrimination? What if the stated preference were related to the religion or religious beliefs of the patient or volunteer? What if it were around lifestyle issues of either the patient or the volunteer?

In addition to potential conflict between the value of allowing autonomy and control to the patient/volunteer versus preventing discrimination to either party, we must also factor in the practical issues of providing good care. Forced matches between patients and volunteers are likely to result in increased potential for less satisfactory care, based on a lack of comfort or ability to interact effectively. Kasengele[4] in a study of hospice providers in New South Wales found that only 9 per cent of volunteers felt they had appropriate skills to work with patients from culturally and linguistically diverse backgrounds.

4 Relationships between patients and volunteers:

Some of the more interesting boundary issues around volunteer involvement develop because of the very good relationships that volunteers can form with patients. Commonly these relationships—when working well—will tend to expand in scope, with the volunteer offering to do more for the patient than is stated in the assignment description of the volunteer. This can include offering to provide personal services outside those normally offered by hospice (shopping, repair work, cleaning services, etc.). It might—in an alternate form—consist of the creation of a romantic relationship between the volunteer and patient or the volunteer and a family member. It might also consist of actions by the patient who feels a strong affection or obligation toward the volunteer—resulting in the offer of a gratuity or gift.

In each these cases the ethical issue for the VSMs is in to what extent the volunteer programme has the right to intrude in personal activities of the volunteer or the patient. Does the volunteer programme have the authority or obligation to say to the patient or volunteer that certain activities are not allowable? And, if so, by what method can the volunteer programme enforce this dictate, especially if the behaviour is initiated by the patient?

5 Relationships between staff and volunteers:

An ethical question for VSMs is whether their own loyalty is to the paid staff of the organization or to its volunteers, and whether they are willing to fight within the organization on behalf of the interests of volunteers. Ellis[5] notes:

In my opinion, we have an ethical dilemma whenever we find ourselves:
- Working around resistance from paid staff (or veteran volunteers) rather than confronting and changing it.
- Seeing that there are no consequences when employees are unsupportive of volunteers and, maybe worse, that there are no rewards for doing a great job with volunteers.
- Accepting restrictions on what volunteers can and can't do that are created under negative, outdated, or otherwise wrong stereotypes about who volunteers are and whether they can be trusted.
- Allowing volunteers to be invisible or of lowest attention on organizational charts, in agency brochures, in annual reports, on Web sites, etc.

6 Staff and volunteer boundaries:

In considering these dilemmas for VSMs, some are further highlighted in exploring boundaries between paid staff and volunteers. It is important that volunteers become an integral and valued part of the hospice team. There are a number of areas, however, where staff and volunteer boundaries may become blurred.

Historically a number of hospices have involved professionals as volunteers and volunteer nurses may be found working alongside paid nurses, often undertaking most of the duties of their paid counterparts. Is it appropriate to recruit some nurses as paid staff but not others? On the other hand, many of these volunteer nurses are employed in other settings and involved in the hospice on a very part-time basis to enable them to further develop skills in palliative care. If volunteer nurses are not supplanting staff roles, could it be considered that they enhance the service offered to patients?

It is not only in nursing, however, where this happens. Often volunteers work alongside staff in very similar roles, for example, in administration. Is this also an inappropriate use of volunteers, or does it strengthen the hospice multidisciplinary team by diversifying skill mix, and motivation?

Yet another challenge for hospices arises as volunteers become more involved over time, often taking on a number of different roles, or offering their services over a number of days. Whilst this undoubtedly adds to the skills and flexibility of the volunteer team, how many hours are too many for a volunteer? When does increasing levels of volunteer involvement highlight the need for additional staff?

In a small organization there may also be complexities where there may be a single post holder, for example, hospice shop managers. In this circumstance, is it ethical to ask volunteers to cover staff holidays and if so should the volunteer be paid?

Conflicts for the individual volunteer

It is not only staff who face such challenges, however, volunteers also face ethical conflicts in performing their volunteer service. These include:

1 Disagreement with organizational values:

Volunteers may hold ethical beliefs that potentially conflict with the values or standards of the hospice programme and indeed with those of the patient and family. Volunteers in hospice may, in fact, be more likely to face such a conflict than volunteers with other programmes. Payne[6] found that religious beliefs were very important or quite important to 71 per cent of hospice volunteers in New Zealand. Such beliefs can easily come into conflict with organizational practices. McMahon[7] discusses the split between the values of sanctity of life and patient autonomy. Zehnder and Royse[8] found, for example, that 37 per cent of volunteers surveyed endorsed the view that there are situations when assisting death may be morally acceptable; 4 per cent had been asked to provide assistance to help a patient end his or her life.

This issue is obviously more critical to hospices are they engage in outreach recruitment to involve volunteers from more diverse cultures and segments of the community (see Crawley and Singer[9]; Kesengele[4], and Taylor and Box[10]).

2 Conflict of loyalty to the patient versus the hospice programme:

One of the overlooked consequences of high levels of volunteer motivation is that it can result in strange patterns of behaviour by volunteers, especially as it relates to loyalty toward the patient versus the volunteer programme (see McCurley[11], for a complete examination of this syndrome). Volunteers must often choose whether to heed what they perceive to be the interests of the patients or the interests of the volunteer programme (as indicated through its policies dictating what the volunteer should and should not do). These competing interests can come into conflict in a number of ways:

◆ The patient expresses a wish for assistance that is not within the boundaries of acceptable service as defined by the hospice programme, but the volunteer wishes to help the patient however they can and so determines to provide the service anyway.

◆ The programme has rules for reporting abusive behaviour by the patient (or a family member) that the volunteer may choose to ignore out of affection for the patient.

Volunteers will face a similar dilemma in determining whether they have a greater loyalty to the patient or to family members when the wishes of these two parties conflict.

Most often, volunteers will tend to resolve all of the above conflicts in favour of the interest of the patient if the volunteer has formed a close personal relationship with the patient. Hospice volunteers may be particularly subject to this syndrome because of their high levels of empathy, which is a primary motivation for their involvement in hospice (see Egbert[12]).

3 Confidentiality of patient information:

All volunteer programmes have rules on confidentiality of patient information. Volunteers usually adhere to these rules, but such adherence is much more difficult in small communities where outside personal relationships are all-pervasive. Volunteers who are known to be assisting a particular patient will be asked by their friends and neighbours (who are also the friends and neighbours of the patient) what is happening with the patient. In this case, the organizational value of protection of the privacy of the patient conflicts with the societal value of sharing information about members of the community.

More serious ethical conflicts around confidentiality can arise when the volunteer has access to information about patient behaviour that may break the law (see McCurley and Ellis[13]). Hospice volunteers with access to patient homes may encounter situations where they are privy to information about the patient or their family members that they may or may not feel comfortable in reporting to the hospice programme, especially if the volunteers is sympathetic to the conduct (such as use of alternative medications or treatment that may not be authorized or legal).

4 Disagreements between the volunteer and the treatment team:

As volunteers become more experienced they will begin to form more opinions about how patients should be treated. Often, this is based on the fact that volunteers may feel they have more experience with both the condition and wishes of the patients than do members of the treatment team—based on their greater degree of contact with the patient. This can be exacerbated if the volunteer does not feel a sense of involvement with the treatment team, either in the sense that they are not listened to by the treatment team or if they do not receive full communication from the treatment team about the basis for decisions being made about the patient. Volunteers may, through loyalty to the patient, decide to resolve their ethical difficulty by not following the guidance of the treatment team or by providing incorrect information to the patient or family members.

Resolving ethical conflict situations

We will divide our suggestions for resolving ethical conflict situations into two parts:

◆ Systemic solutions
◆ Individual situations

Systemic solutions

The following will enhance the ability of the VSMs to deal with ethical conflicts:

1 Develop standards and procedures that relate to common ethical conflict situations:

Many of the conflict situations we examined earlier could be addressed by clear standards of practice. As an example, consider the following standards for interaction with patients, carers, and families produced by Volunteering Victoria[14]:

4. Interaction with patients, carers, and families

In all instances, the onus of responsibility to communicate the boundaries of the volunteer role resides with the manager of volunteers. Volunteers are only required to carry out the duties of their role specified in a written position description authorized by the manager of volunteers. Volunteers need to be aware that:

- They may only undertake or assume responsibility for any duties specified in writing by the manager of volunteers or agreed to in consultation with the manager of volunteers.
- Any requests from patients, carers, and families to perform activities outside the volunteer position description needs to be referred to the manager of volunteers for consideration and approval.
- Any perceived opportunities to improve service delivery can be discussed with the manager of volunteers or the interdisciplinary team, and only enacted with organization approval.

In the event that a volunteer is given a direction or duty that the volunteer feels is inappropriate or does not feel equipped to comply with, the volunteer can:

- Decline to perform the direction or duty and provide reasons why this is appropriate.
- Request that alternative arrangements be made to fulfil a particular direction or duty.

As the programme develops a history of volunteers encountering ethical issues appropriate standards should be developed to indicate the values of the hospice programme and to provide direction to the volunteers.

While formal procedures such as that given earlier are important, it is also critical to develop informal rules. This is especially true in boundary areas related to relationships with patients. Adopt and communicate to all volunteers a 'non-abandonment' policy regarding patient needs that they encounter that do not fall into the normal work of the programme. Urge volunteers to bring these needs to you and let them know that you will work to find some way of meeting the needs, usually through referral to another agency. Stress to the volunteer that the programme will not intend to 'abandon' the patient. It is crucial to maintain open communication with the volunteers regarding these issues, and it is equally crucial to get them to know that you are on the same side as they are—each of you wants to do what it takes to help the patient. If a volunteer ever gets the impression that the programme doesn't 'care' about the patients, they will be much more likely simply to act on their own and they will eventually be likely to stop volunteering.

2 Engage in scenario-based interviewing and training:

Many ethical dilemmas are not susceptible to easy rules and simple procedures. Volunteers may not easily realize why they feel troubled by some issues or what they would do when confronted by them.

One solution to this is to utilize more realistic role-playing scenarios during interviewing and training of volunteers. These scenarios allow both the volunteer and the managers to think about and work through complex situations.

A. Think about past problems that your volunteers have encountered. Select one that has some of the following characteristics:

- Worries you and might occur again.
- Has no clear 'right' answer or represents a conflict of ethical interests and values.

- ◆ A volunteer might be likely to rush to their own 'right' answer to the problem.
- ◆ A volunteer might have difficulty in dealing with the subject matter.
- ◆ A volunteer might have difficulty in dealing with the interpersonal relations involved in the situation.

B. Briefly outline:

- ◆ Main facts and characters
- ◆ Basic 'dilemma'
- ◆ Key elements
- ◆ 'Wrong' responses

C. Further develop this situation into an interviewing scenario:

- ◆ Description of basic setting to be given to volunteer
- ◆ Characters involved
- ◆ Key starting questions
- ◆ Secondary twists and complexities

These same scenarios can be utilized for discussion in volunteer training sessions.

3 Create volunteer discussion groups:

Many of the difficulties around ethical dilemmas for the volunteer can be avoided by providing the volunteer with opportunities to discuss their feelings and explore acceptable solutions with others. Some of this discussion can occur between the volunteer and their designated supervisor, but the volunteer may find it difficult to 'confess' that they are tempted to break organizational rules. Volunteers will be more likely to admit these feelings to other volunteers and then to talk openly about possible solutions to their ethical conflicts. Volunteers will also be more likely not to feel guilty about these feelings, a condition that can lead to stress and burnout. Volunteers often cite expanded contact and communication with other volunteers as valuable to them[15]. Siebold, et al.[16] found that 49 per cent of surveyed hospice volunteers listed 'more contact with other volunteers' as a desired form of support.

In addition to giving volunteers a forum for raising ethical questions, these discussion groups are an excellent venue for utilizing experienced volunteers as group leaders.

4 Foster inclusion and involvement of volunteers in hospice staff teams:

Volunteers who feel they are active and productive members of the overall hospice team are more likely to understand and adhere to the values of the hospice programme. Conversely, volunteers who do not feel bonded to the hospice are more likely to follow their own inclinations when faced with a conflict situation. This involvement should go beyond volunteer simply being informed about what is happening; they should be allowed the opportunity to provide input and to fully discuss the situation of the patient.

Andersson and Ohlen[17] explain this concept:

Where hospices provided structured volunteer support, an essential part in promoting a favourable reception from staff was the information session and follow-up that took place.

Good information gives a sense of being on the team. However, even when a volunteer was positive about the information they had received, there may have been a lingering desire for deeper contact, such as getting an opportunity'to sit down a little more and talk things through'.

Individual situations

The suggestions above will assist in avoiding or managing ethical conflicts in general. What we will discuss next are some steps in dealing with particular ethical situations as they arise.

The decision-making process in the following paragraphs is intended to guide the VSM as they think through a particular situation, and is intended to ensure that the decision that is made is one that accurately reflects the ethical values of the hospice programme and one that will cohere with future decisions.

As you consider what action to take in a situation involving an ethical conflict or dilemma think about the following:

1 What are the facts in this situation? Do you have all the relevant information? Do you have information from all sides? Is this information reliable and unbiased? Have you considered how various stakeholders may interpret the information differently?

2 Who are the various stakeholders and what do they have to lose/gain in the situation? What rights are in conflict? Which of their values are in conflict? (Stakeholders may include the patient and family members, volunteers, the hospice programme, and even the community in general.)

3 What ethical principles or values underlie the situation? How do these values differ among the various stakeholders? Are there priorities among those values? Are there key values of the hospice programme that must be upheld in this situation?

4 What decision will resolve this current situation and what principles/values is the decision based upon? Whose interests are best supported by this decision? Whose interests are lost?

5 Who should be involved in making this decision so that all interests are fairly represented?

6 How well will this decision carry to other similar situations involving the same principles/values? Will we be willing to apply the same decision to those situations? Would we be willing to apply this decision to our own actions?

7 What actions will we need to take in the future to uphold this decision?

8 Would you be willing to explain this decision to the media? To your co-workers? To children?

This process will make it more likely that the decision reached will be correct and more acceptable to all parties, both present and future.

Conclusion

Beneath the surface of the involvement of and support provided by volunteers in hospices lies a web of relationships and a range of philosophies. VSMs face the responsibility of reconciling these varying interests, understanding that the smooth operation of the volunteer programme requires integrating a variety of beliefs, values, and ethical standards held by volunteers, patients, hospice staff, and others. These values are significant to their holders, and this is especially true in the case of hospice volunteers whose beliefs are integral to their motivation and involvement in hospices. The philosophical questions and dilemmas faced by hospice volunteers are as troubling as some of the practical medical issues. Effective VSMs will understand the need to support not only volunteers, but also hospice staff and the organization itself, as they confront many of the difficult ethical decisions faced in their daily work.

References

1 Association for Volunteer Administration. (2005). Professional Ethics in Volunteer Administration. www.cvacert.org/documents/ProfessionalEthicsinVolunteerAdministration-2006.pdf

2 British Columbia Hospice Palliative Care Association. (2007). *Volunteer Standards for Hospice Palliative Care in British Columbia*. Vancouver, BC, British Columbia Hospice Palliative Care Association.

3 Merrill, M. (accessed 10 April 2008). Leadership and ethics in volunteer management. www.merrillassociates.net/topic/2002/04/leadership-and-ethics-volunteer-management

4 Kasengele, P. (2003). *Palliative Care for a Culturally Diverse Community in Wentworth Area Health Service*. NSW, Australia, Wentworth Area Health Service.

5 Ellis, S. (2007, accessed 10 April 2008). The moral obligation of volunteer recruitment promises. www.energizeinc.com/hot/2007/07oct.html

6 Payne, S. (2001). The role of volunteers in hospice bereavement support in New Zealand. *Palliative Medicine* 15, 107–115.

7 McMahon, R. (2003). An ethical dilemma in a hospice setting. *Palliative and Support Care* 4, 79–87.

8 Zehnder, P. and Royse, D. (1999). Attitudes toward assisted suicide: a survey of hospice volunteers. *Hospice Journal* 14(2), 49–63.

9 Crawley, L. and Singer, M. (March 2007). *Racial, cultural and ethnic factors affecting the quality of end-of-life care in California: supplemental materials*. Oakland, CA, California Healthcare Foundation.

10 Taylor, T. and Box, M. (1999). *Multicultural Palliative Care Guidelines*. Deakin West ACT, Palliative Care Australia.

11 McCurley, S. (1994, accessed 10 April 2008). Utilizing role-playing scenarios in volunteer interviewing. nationalserviceresources.org/filemanager/download/708/roleplay_interviews.pdf

12 Egbert, N. and Parrott, R. (2003). Empathy and social support for the terminally ill: implications for recruiting and retaining hospice and hospital volunteers. *Communication Studies* 54, 18–34.

13 McCurley, S. and Ellis, S. (2004). Confidentiality and the Volunteer Situation. *e-Volunteerism*, June-September 2004. www.e-volunteerism.com

14 Volunteering Victoria. (April 2007). *Strengthening Palliative Care: Palliative Care Volunteer Standards*. Melbourne VIC, Victoria Government Department of Human Services.

15 Claxton-Oldfield, S. and Claxton-Oldfield, J. (2007). The impact of volunteering in hospice palliative care. *American Journal of Hospice and Palliative Care* 24, 259–263.

16 Seibold, D., Rossi, S., Berteotti, C., Soprych, S., and McQuillan, L. (1987). Volunteer involvement in a hospice care programme: an examination of motives, activities. *American Journal of Hospice and Palliative Care* **4**, 43–54.

17 Andersson, B. and Ohlen, J. (2005). Being a hospice volunteer. *Palliative Medicine* **19**, 602–608.

Chapter 11

Volunteers working in a bereavement service

Jenny Osterfield

Do bereaved people need help and, if so, what intervention is helpful? What happens to the survivors when a person dies? No one person's reaction to loss is the same as another's but the pain of grief is universal, and many of the experiences surrounding death and bereavement are universal. When planning a bereavement service, these fundamental questions need to be addressed. Dr Colin Murray Parkes speaks of bereavement as having a detrimental effect upon physical and mental health[1].

Help for the bereaved should be deeply rooted in the culture and community in which it is being experienced. In Western society today, we avoid talking about death and we have largely abandoned the rituals with which our ancestors dealt with death. It is possible to reach adult life without ever having first-hand experience of death or a funeral. The sympathy of relatives and friends is all too often aimed at preventing rather than promoting the expression of grief so that open expression of pain and sadness is usually discouraged.

Different cultures have different ways of coping with grief; what is expected and considered normal in one culture is taboo in another. In some cultures, the whole community is involved but in others the families are left isolated and alone. In East Africa, for instance, death is seen as a natural part of life; people seldom die in hospital but on mats on the floor of their homes and the grief of the family is shared by the whole community.

Whatever our culture or society, the pain of bereavement needs to find appropriate expression. There is a universal need to talk about the death, to go over again and again the events associated with the loss, to accept it, and find a meaning to carry on with life. The bereaved need permission to grieve. Fortunately, most people do get through their grief with the support of their family and friends, but for those who need help, hospices are in an ideal position to provide it. The question for the hospice or palliative care service is: 'Is there a need for a bereavement service?' and if one is operated, the question for the Bereavement Service Coordinator is: 'Where do I begin and who should be involved?'

No single approach

A bereavement service must be wanted. It must be designed to meet real, identified needs[2]. What are the needs of the bereaved? Befriending, counselling, support groups, practical help, social clubs, memorial services?

The list is a long one and will be influenced by the ethnic, cultural, and social groups to which people belong and whether any bereavement support already exists in their area. Personal research of the services provided by other British hospices showed that many different approaches were used with priority being given to opportunities for the bereaved to share their grief in a one-to-one relationship. In many cases, volunteers were being used to provide this support.

Research carried out by the Bereavement Care Standards U.K. Project estimated that 80 per cent of bereavement support in Britain is delivered by the voluntary sector (that is to say, non-statutory, unpaid, and charity-funded) and 90 per cent of it by volunteers[3].

The successful placing of volunteers to support the terminally ill and their families in their own homes over many years led naturally to the decision to use volunteers as providers of bereavement care. It was important, however, to be clear about the role of the bereavement volunteers and what they are equipped and can be trained to do[4].

Volunteers: a link to the community

Why are volunteers rather than professionals so widely involved in providing bereavement care in British hospices? If volunteers are drawn from a wide variety of backgrounds and life experiences, they not only represent the community but provide a link to it. Volunteers demonstrate that bereavement is not a mental or physical illness but a normal reaction to the loss of someone close. 'The widespread involvement of volunteers underlines the concept that grief is natural. Volunteers are ordinary people and carry none of the stigma attached to mental health services, counselling, or therapy'[4].

Volunteers fulfill many different roles within the hospice and may continue to work in these areas in addition to supporting bereaved families. Their roles may include working on the wards, with the community volunteer team, in day care, or as a driver, hairdresser, or lay chaplain. Volunteers working on the wards may develop the kind of supportive relationships that make them the best person to support a family member after bereavement[5].

> A volunteer working on the ward shared with a family the powerlessness of watching the lingering death of father and husband. His wife struggled with her pain and distress at watching the suffering of her husband and confided to the volunteer that she did not think she could ever live without him. After he died she did not respond at first to offers of support feeling, as she told us 'that I have to put on a brave face'. Now, with her grief still raw and bubbling to the surface, she is responding well to help from the same volunteer who befriended her on the ward and who remembers her husband and all that he and the family suffered. She does not have to pretend any more.

Volunteers are unpaid but they are not amateurs! With careful selection, the right training, supervision, and support, they are ideally placed to offer families bereavement support.

The selection minefield

Who makes a good bereavement volunteer, and how do we recognize them? Unlike many other forms of voluntary work, bereavement counselling rarely brings immediate satisfaction. We are asking volunteers often to visit someone they have not met before and to make this visit on their own. The family wants their dead returned to them, and the effort of talking about their loss is exceedingly distressing and they may be reluctant to communicate[2]. Volunteers have to be able to stay with depression and pain through weeks or months without seeing much change or becoming too discouraged. They have to be comfortable with the sharing of painful feelings, tears, and anger. They have to be able to listen without giving advice.

Such people need to have sensitivity, warmth, common sense, courage, and realism. They must be good listeners, non-judgemental, and able to cope with the anxieties and fears of the bereaved. Bereavement counselling can sometimes reawaken the counsellor's own painful feelings of loss, and volunteers need to be self-aware and accepting of supervision.

Experience has shown that seeking new bereavement volunteers from amongst volunteers and staff who have already been working in other disciplines in the hospice for at least 6 months has many advantages. They have been exposed to the philosophy of palliative care and have had experience of working with death and dying before they apply to work with the bereaved. In addition to the interview process insights about the suitability of the applicant can be sought from the Voluntary Services Manager (VSM) or their line manager/team leader. This reduces the risk of selecting volunteers unsuited to the task and is an ideal method of recruitment if few volunteers are required, or are additions to an already established team. If larger numbers are needed, it is unlikely that enough volunteers will come forward in-house to make this method of recruitment viable. In this case, recruitment will need to be on a much wider basis through advertisements in the community and word of mouth. A good method of recruitment is to offer a training course on loss and bereavement to the local community. This usually attracts many different people. At the end of the course, any participants who are interested in becoming bereavement volunteers are invited to apply.

Many people are drawn to this type of work because of personal experience but not all are suitable. Some may unconsciously be searching for a way of working through their own grief or loss. It can sometimes be difficult to distinguish between potential helpers and those needing help for themselves. Doing this work often brings to the surface past losses or difficulties. If these have not been sufficiently resolved, training and supervision sessions risk becoming personal therapy for individual volunteers[4]. Unresolved grief can linger for many years, and it is important to look for signs of continuing difficulties at the interview.

The selection of bereavement volunteers needs to be as thorough as possible. It is not only the service but also the volunteers and their families who have to live with the stress and tension, which can be caused by an unwise decision[2]. If there is any uncertainty as to suitability it is better to reject a volunteer than to take them on for this type of work. Mistakes can lead to a lack of confidence in the service by the bereaved and feelings of failure, anger, and disappointment in the volunteer.

The application form

Selection should be a two-way process enabling potential volunteers to find out what is involved in the role of helping bereaved people, as well as enabling judgements to be made about their suitability. It is beneficial to invite those interested in volunteering to attend an informal discussion where they have the opportunity to meet with active volunteers, learn about what is involved, and ask questions.

Those who decide to proceed should be given a simple application form to complete. The purpose of this form is to ask them to think about their motives for wanting to work with bereaved people and their understanding of what is involved.

Application forms should request much the same information as applications for other volunteer roles, but with some important additions focused on experience of loss:

- Name, address, and telephone number.
- Date of birth.
- Current driving licence or any transport difficulties.
- Details of current occupation or hospice voluntary work.
- Any experience, training, or qualifications relevant to working with bereaved people.
- Brief details, including dates, of any major personal loss including bereavement, redundancy, divorce or separation, and serious illness.
- Name, address, and telephone number of one or two referees who can vouch for their suitability for this type of work.
- Short (400-word) essay: 'What makes you interested in helping bereaved people? What is the role of a bereavement volunteer and what qualities and skills do you feel you have that would enable you to do this kind of work?'

The completed application form will enable a judgement to be made as to whether the applicant should be called forward for interview.

A two-tiered model for selection

A most effective method of selecting volunteers for bereavement work is to approach selection in two stages; an individual interview followed by a group case study. Applicants are usually nervous at interview and judgements made about their suitability may then be checked out as the case study progresses. It is helpful to have two interviewers as this enables a more objective and professional approach and allows a joint decision about the applicant to be made.

It is important to prepare for and structure the interviews to focus on:

- Motivation for wanting to work with the bereaved.
- Interests and beliefs.
- Attitudes and prejudices.
- Past losses and crises and how these were handled.
- How they support and sustain themselves.

- Their own family.
- Empathy, openness, and sensitivity.
- Intelligence and willingness to learn.
- Any relevant past experience.
- Accepting of supervision.
- Ability to work in a group. Interviewers also need to be alert for non-verbal communication and any emotional undercurrents. Following interview, all applicants are then asked back to participate in a group case study. Cases and scenarios are presented to the group for discussion or, alternatively, the group is asked to take part in a 'sculpt', an experiential learning technique, if this technique is known. In either case, the attitudes, opinions, and skills of the applicants give the interviewers valuable insights as to their suitability for working with the bereaved.

Selection needs to be ongoing throughout initial training and the probationary period.

Which training course?

Volunteers bring with them the individual qualities for which they have been selected, their life experiences, and their own tested ways of handling crises and disappointments. The challenge is how to train them without de-skilling them or devaluing the personal contributions that they bring[2]. Volunteers need initial preparation to work with the bereaved, and ongoing training helps them to build and develop their skills. Initial training should cover:

- Knowledge—to acquire an understanding of loss and bereavement, theories, and models of grief.
- Skills—practice in basic counselling skills.
- Self-awareness—awareness of how their own feelings and experiences may help or hinder the counselling process.

The course needs to be a balance of theory and practical with role-plays and experiential exercises so that theory is constantly demonstrated in practice. An average course will take 40–60 hours and may need to be run on an annual basis. A course of this nature is a huge commitment and can present difficulties with financial, time, and venue constraints. It is more easily achieved with larger numbers of participants who can benefit from the varied interests and experiences of the group. The experience of shared training with other bereavement agencies in the area can be useful and may build worthwhile bridges for the future. Some British hospices share training with Cruse Bereavement Care (a nationwide bereavement service in the United Kingdom staffed by volunteers), which cuts down on the workload and is beneficial to both organizations. Cruse has excellent trainers, hospices have good venues and support services, and the volunteers benefit from being with a large and varied group. At the end of the course, the bereavement volunteers receive additional hospice sessions to cover the systems, paperwork, confidentiality, supervision, and other related issues particular to the hospice bereavement service. In Britain, an excellent initial training course has been produced by Cruse Bereavement Care UK and Help the Hospices with well-researched and evaluated sessions, handouts, and notes[6].

Most volunteers find the commitment and sacrifice of giving up so much time to initial training well worth it. Some volunteers have described their experiences of initial training as 'life-changing', 'I find the skills work so well on my friends', 'I used to give advice but now I never do', 'my husband and I don't argue as much now'.

What's in a name?

The volunteers have completed their training and are ready to start their probation, but what should they be called?

The advantage of involving volunteers to support the bereaved is that they are not health-care professionals but ordinary people. People who are grieving may know that they are not suffering mental or physical illness but a normal reaction to the loss of someone close. The word 'counsellor' may wrongly imply the need for therapeutic intervention or, alternatively, that the volunteer is trained to a higher level. It is important to choose a name for the team which gives the right message.

In recent years, there has been a debate in the Britain as to the use of the word 'counsellor' for those trained to work with grief. The truth is that bereavement often acts as a catalyst for the resurfacing of unresolved emotional difficulties from the past and over time many bereavement counsellors seek additional training, knowledge, and skills.

Volunteer teams in British hospice bereavement services are called by different names, amongst them 'bereavement support workers', 'bereavement visitors', 'befrienders', 'bereavement counsellors', and 'skilled helpers'. A group of newly trained volunteers who were asked what they wished to be called opted for 'bereavement volunteers' which they felt was a good compromise.

Unlike other hospice volunteers, the identification badges of the bereavement volunteers do not give their surnames. They are known to their clients by their first names and may only be contacted through the Bereavement Service Coordinator. This is to protect them from unsolicited telephone calls or visits from bereaved people who often become distressed and lonely, especially in the evenings and at weekends.

Launched: the probationary period

The volunteer is trained and ready to help their first bereaved person. It is important that they fully understand what is expected of them and what their boundaries are. Guidelines are issued to all bereavement volunteers along with their confidentiality document to sign. The guidelines set out the particular details of working within the bereavement service, what commitment is expected, supervision and support, any required paperwork regarding client visits, how to claim expenses, disciplinary and complaints procedures, and any other issues relevant to the service.

New bereavement volunteers are given one case to start with and after their first visit receive one-to-one supervision either by telephone or face-to-face. In addition to this they attend monthly supervision meetings in a group with other volunteers who have different levels of expertise. This is helpful for them to debrief on their feelings, usually of nervousness, their musings about whether the visit was helpful for the client and any difficulties. Affirmation and reassurance are extremely important. It is beneficial for the coordinator or supervisor to have an open-door policy for bereavement volunteers to contact them about a client at any time. New volunteers will often wish to talk through each visit for the first few times until they become more confident and understand the usefulness of their monthly group supervision.

Probation normally lasts for 6 months but is dependent on the volunteer having sufficient exposure to clients during that period. The number of clients is not as important as the number of contacts. Probationers are treated in the same way as the other bereavement volunteers but their work is monitored more closely. They also attend ongoing training and team meetings. Probation is ended when both the supervisor and volunteer feel that the time is right. The selection process continues until the period of probation has ended.

It is important to allocate cases to probationers at the right skills level if possible. Beginners trying to help cases of abnormal grief or complicated family dynamics may feel unable to cope. Regular monthly supervision, preferably in small mixed-expertise groups, is vital for all bereavement volunteers.

The supervisor as 'enabler'

Volunteers who work with the bereaved need supervision. They need a safe forum where they are encouraged to explore their way of working with clients and look at any reawakened memories of personal losses or difficulties. The primary purpose of supervision is to provide support, ensure accountability, and that boundaries are being maintained, and to enhance and develop skills[3]. The initial training course, together with any ongoing courses, should cover the formal education responsibilities of the service. Supervisors fill in gaps on knowledge and make practical what was once 'head'-knowledge and must now become working-knowledge[7]. Supervision safeguards the well-being of the client, ensuring that his/her needs are being met, and facilitates the professional and personal development of the volunteer. Volunteers will have uniquely different qualities, styles, and ways of working; the supervisor acts as an enabler for these gifts to be used to the best advantage with clients.

Supervision is achieved in a small monthly mixed-expertise group where the volunteers are exposed to a variety of different cases and styles of working. This supervision is mandatory with provision being made for holidays and illness. Easy access to the supervisor at other times is also essential, as has been stressed already, as volunteers may occasionally feel the need to talk if they are struggling with a difficult case or personal issues. In addition, they attend an individual annual supervision and work appraisal, which gives them an opportunity to explore issues of personal development, ongoing training needs, and discuss any difficulties. Volunteers look forward to supervision and most say that they benefit from the time spent with their peers and find the case discussions interesting and helpful.

Supervisors should be counsellors experienced in working with loss and bereavement who have undertaken a course in how to supervise. It is also expected that the supervisor will also be supervised and their work and role be monitored[3]. Wherever possible, an external supervisor should be appointed. The question of who should supervise the bereavement volunteers may be governed by financial constraints so that the Bereavement Service Coordinator may fulfil this role along with the roles of trainer and manager of the service.

Volunteers working with clients

How many cases should a volunteer be given? Pressure of referrals to the service should never be passed on to the volunteers. The time that they are able to give to this work varies enormously according to their personal commitments. Volunteers are allocated one client and take on additional cases after discussion of complexity, frequency of visits, their own availability, and other considerations. Most volunteers handle two cases concurrently.

Bereavement services allocate cases in different ways. In some hospices, volunteers are the first people to have contact with the bereaved but this may present dangers in exposing volunteers to inappropriate referrals, complex cases, or hazardous situations. If the client's first contact is with an experienced counsellor, nurse, or supervisor, this can be avoided. The insights gained into a client's difficulties and past history provide invaluable assistance in the appropriate allocation of cases and allow complex cases to be handled by a more experienced counsellor. It also provides a vehicle for the filtering of inappropriate referrals where there may be a need to refer on to the psychological or psychiatric services or to the client's medical practitioner. Such invaluable information and insights are best provided by the 'care team' members in the hospice, nurses, doctors, social workers, and others who have cared for the patient, possibly both at home and in the hospice, and met many members of the family.

This first interview with the client, which may be at home or in the hospice, also gives an opportunity for their grief reaction to be 'normalized'. The strong emotions experienced in bereavement can prompt feelings of 'going mad' and when reassurance is given often, no further support or intervention is necessary. The support offered by the service and the role of the bereavement volunteer is also explained, enabling clients to make an informed choice about acceptance.

All are encouraged to return to the hospice to meet their bereavement befriender, but there are many cases when this may not be possible or desirable and support is then given through home visits. Whether at hospice or home, the frequency of visits is dependent on the degree of help needed. It is usual for visits to be more frequent at first with increasingly longer gaps as the client feels more able to cope. The number of visits is not set and the management of each case is monitored in supervision to ensure that the support given is enabling and empowering for the client and that dependency is not being created. Endings need to be managed sensitively and can be difficult for both the client and the bereavement volunteer.

Compassion fatigue

Folk wisdom tells us that when the waves crash in, no matter how hard the rock it will erode over time.[8]

Continually witnessing pain and grief can have a cumulative emotional impact, which can make it difficult for volunteers to continue to offer support[3]. In some cases, the cause may be obvious and related to the particular bereavement they are supporting but in other cases, it is less obvious. It may have nothing to do with their work but with outside events, home and family, friends, hospice staff, or other volunteers. These can upset and interfere with the support systems they have come to rely on[9]. Such feelings may make a volunteer feel overwhelmed, insecure, or ashamed. It is important that volunteers are offered emotional support in addition to supervision.

Time spent in supervision should centre on the work with the client. It may pick up emotional difficulties for a volunteer in handling a particular case, but it is not the place to give attention to the needs of volunteers in fulfilling this role. An open-door policy for support is important as well as keeping a watchful eye on the team in an attempt to avoid casualties. Caring for each other and peer support is also encouraged. It is sometimes, but not always, possible to predict when problems may occur. Emotional involvement and over-identification with clients, feelings of anger, spiritual distress, depression, unusual sensitivity, or irritability are all signs that something may be amiss. In such instances, volunteers are given the opportunity for confidential counselling and support from the staff support counsellor appointed from an outside agency. There is no stigma attached to 'resting' from bereavement work for a while. A few volunteers take time out during a personal crisis or difficulty such as illness and family difficulties. A gentle easing back into casework is facilitated when the volunteer feels ready.

The support offered by the hospice will only be useful if volunteers take on the responsibility of caring for themselves and are aware of their own weaknesses and vulnerabilities. It is also important to foster a good team spirit with opportunities for humour and a pervading sense of hope. The occasional social event provides an ideal opportunity for this.

Safety: whose responsibility is it?

A difficult bereavement visit was a forceful reminder of the importance of having a safety policy in place for home visits. The house was in an isolated spot, the bereaved gentleman appeared very strange and was accompanied by an evil-tempered dog. It soon became apparent that discussing his bereavement was the least of his intentions. Extrication was difficult and frightening.

Inclusion of discussion on issues of personal safety, potential dangers, and common sense practical guidelines should form part of the volunteer's initial training course, with reminders annually. Hospices need to take all reasonable precautions to ensure the safety of their volunteers but responsibility for personal safety has to ultimately rest with the person making the visit.

Box 11.1 Guidelines on safety for volunteers

- The volunteer should always let family or hospice know where they intend to go.
- The volunteer should let family or hospice know the expected duration of the visit.
- The volunteer must remember to advise the hospice if plans are altered.
- Safety guidelines must be issued to all bereavement volunteers, highlighting the importance of trusting their instincts and judgements and using their common sense. Volunteers should never feel pressurized into making a home visit if they have any doubts, and if they feel uncomfortable in any situation they should make an excuse and leave immediately.
- Volunteers should be asked to report any incidents, however small, to the hospice. Training needs to include skills in the diffusion of anger and threatening behaviour.

Ongoing training

The initial training course gives the volunteer the essential basic knowledge and skills to work with bereaved people. Practical experience of working with different clients, supervision, and ongoing training will increase these skills. The need for additional training is identified by both the supervisor and the volunteers who are encouraged to identify their own gaps in knowledge and skills. Opportunities are given for volunteers to research and present topics of interest to share with their peers. Case studies, role-plays, brainstorming, videos, experiential exercises, and 'sculpting' are all used. Sculpting is a particularly helpful technique used to provide insights into relationships, alliances, and feelings in family or group dynamics. Involvement and participation by the volunteers increases their knowledge of theories, their self-awareness, and confidence. Ongoing training is done in-house on a quarterly basis when the whole team has an opportunity to get together. It is combined with a brief administrative period when hospice and issues pertaining to the bereavement service and volunteers are dealt with. These quarterly meetings also foster a team spirit by providing a regular opportunity for sharing and peer support.

Volunteers are also encouraged to read and provide items of interest for circulation from newspaper or magazine articles, book, or film reviews.

Hospice bereavement care: a proactive approach

Unlike many other agencies in the community, hospices have the opportunity to be proactive in offering help, support, and information to the bereaved. We do not have to wait until problems occur to give help. It is important to keep a balance between offering initial support and making a family feel that they are unable to cope. All bereaved families are given the opportunity of a routine visit 6 weeks to 2 months following the death. This visit is then made by the Bereavement Service Coordinator who is able to make an assessment of needs. Allocation to a volunteer in then made if further help is requested at this stage. Bereaved people who are considered more at risk or vulnerable are targeted earlier through a well-researched bereavement profile questionnaire. This gives details of the death, the family relationships, known social support networks, and other predisposing factors[10]. It is completed, as has been explained earlier, by the multidisciplinary care team and discussed at the weekly ward clinical meeting with the Bereavement Service Coordinator who is able to make an assessment of risk. Any one who has been identified as being at risk of having difficulties are offered support at an earlier stage through a telephone call by a volunteer.

Hospice bereavement care is offered within the context of palliative care. The nursing and pastoral care teams who care for families in the period leading up to the death often know them well. At this time, the needs of the patient take precedence and relatives will often deny their own feelings of grief in order to keep control and continue to care for the dying person[5]. Involvement of the bereavement service is only requested if complex issues, such as multiple prior bereavements, are identified. Bereavement volunteers will give in-depth support to these family members and occasionally to patients who are grieving in anticipation of their own deaths. In such cases, the volunteers receive additional one-to-one supervision.

Once the death has occurred, the bereaved family are referred to the bereavement service for ongoing support. All families are offered two opportunities to attend bereavement afternoons or evenings staffed by a team of nurses and volunteers. The aim of these events is to give an opportunity for families to return to the hospice, to 'normalize' grief, and to enable bereaved people to meet each other.

Volunteers who are not bereavement volunteers, help at these events by welcoming families back to the hospice, serving refreshments, and making them feel at home. They are not regarded as bereavement counsellors but are given training in listening skills and basic theories of loss and bereavement. Because families usually like to see the nurses who cared for their loved ones and helped the relatives at the time of the death some nurses also attend. Such events offer an opportunity to meet and share with other people who have been bereaved in a welcoming environment with which they are familiar. However, as has been noted, not everyone wants to return to the hospice.

Help for bereaved children

Many British hospices help bereaved children by offering a service especially tailored to their needs. Some have appointed separate coordinators for adult and children's bereavement services. Many of the children's services also help bereaved children in the local community and are run jointly with community services. Children benefit greatly by meeting other children who are bereaved and group work is often offered in preference to individual counselling.

Surviving parents, families, close friends, or teachers with whom the child has a good relationship are usually the best people to support grieving children. Information on how children grieve and support for families before and after the death are offered but there are some occasions when children need individual support. Volunteers working with children should have experience working with bereaved adults before undertaking additional training. This training needs to cover the way children and adolescents grieve, creative ways of working with children, and resources that can be used. Criminal record checks are necessary under the U.K. Child Protection Act for any team member who offers one-to-one support to children.

The hospice bereavement service: a community resource

The hospice bereavement service is a resource for the community offering information about grief, education, and training to professionals and workshops to community and faith groups. Volunteers play a large part in 'normalizing' the process of grieving in the community and in helping society to see that there is a need to support those who are suffering after the death of someone close.

Bereavement volunteers: the last word

The last word must come from the bereavement volunteers themselves. They admit that the going is often hard at times but the reward of seeing someone eventually move on with their lives cannot be measured. They say that they mostly 'enjoy' their work but comment that they are not sure that 'enjoy' is quite the right word!

References

1 Parkes, C.M. (1991). *Bereavement: Studies of Grief in Adult Life,* (2nd edition). London, Penguin.

2 Earnshaw-Smith, E. and Yorkstone, P. (1986). *Setting up and Running a Bereavement Service.* London, St. Christopher's Hospice.

3 *Standards for bereavement care in the UK.* (2001). Bereavement Care Standards: UK Project. (Available from London Bereavement Network, 356 Holloway Road, London N7 6PA; also at: www.bereavement.org.uk)

4 Relf, M. (1998). Involving volunteers in bereavement counselling. *European Journal of Palliative Care* 5(2), 61–5.

5 Parkes, C.M. (1998). Bereavement. In *Oxford Textbook of Palliative Medicine*, (ed. D. Doyle, G.W. Hanks, and N. MacDonald). Oxford University Press.

6 Faulkner, A. and Wallbank, S. (1998). *Bereavement Counselling.* Help the Hospices and Cruse Bereavement Care. (Available from Help the Hospices, 34–44 Britannia Street, London, WC1X 9JG.)

7 Carroll, M. (1996). *Counselling Supervision.* London, Cassell.

8 Bowman, T. (1999). Promoting resiliency in those who do bereavement work. *Lifeline, Journal of the National Association of Bereavement Services,* 27, Spring.

9 Parkes, C.M. (1986). The caregivers griefs. *Journal of Palliative Care* 1(2), 5–6.

10 Parkes, C.M. (1990). Risk factors in bereavement: Implications for the prevention and treatment of pathological grief. *Psychiatric Annals,* 20(6), 310.

Recommended reading

Jeffrey, D. (2002). *Teaching Palliative Care, a Practical Guide.* Abingdon, Radcliffe Medical Press.

Walshe, C. (1997). Whom to help? An exploration of the assessment of grief. *International Journal of Palliative Nursing* 3(3), 132–7.

Faulkner, A. (1998). *Working with Bereaved People.* London, Harcourt Brace.

Chapter 12

Volunteers in a children's hospice

Ros Scott

Children and families benefit significantly from the added value that volunteers bring to children's hospices. Complementing the skills and expertise of the staff team, volunteers have much to offer in terms of skills, experience, and time. Their involvement helps to ensure a truly holistic approach to care.

In the same way as in adult hospices, however, volunteers do not just happen and the development of a service requires careful planning and commitment. Volunteers are entitled to expect the same supervision, support, and guidance as paid staff but this must be delivered through a very different approach. The management task, as can be seen in Chapter 3, is considerable and is not ideally added to an already busy professional role. The secret of effective management is that the service is organized with great precision, but is portrayed to the volunteers in a relaxed and friendly way.

An introduction to children's hospices

Children's hospices provide specialist palliative respite care and terminal care to children and young people with a life-limiting or life-threatening condition[1]. Care extends to the whole family, including parents, siblings, and grandparents and may be offered in the hospice or in the child's home. This care also extends beyond the death of the child into bereavement support for the family. Children of all ages may be cared for from babies to young people in their twenties. Some children's hospices have developed special units to offer such care to young adults extending into thirties and forties.

Within a children's hospice, as in adult hospices, the emphasis is on living and helping to make the most of the time children and young people have left. Hospices are well equipped with play facilities for children, and there are many opportunities to take part in activities or just to have some quiet time and relaxation. Multi-sensory rooms, jacuzzis, hydrotherapy pools, teenage 'dens', and soft playrooms are just some of the specialist facilities found in a children's hospice.

When children are first diagnosed with a life-limiting condition or when curative treatment becomes unsuccessful, many families experience fear, isolation, and a huge sense of loss. As the child's condition deteriorates, families find themselves under enormous strain. Simple things such as a good night's sleep, shopping, or even taking children to the park become difficult, if not impossible. Family life necessarily revolves round the needs of the affected child and siblings often cannot lead normal lives and, in many cases, have a significant role to play in the care of their brother or sister.

Because of the genetic nature of some conditions, families may have more than one affected child, requiring complex and continual care. Most children's hospices offer accommodation for parents and siblings in order that the whole family can spend time together and benefit from the support offered during their stay. They also offer opportunities to meet and form bonds with other parents and siblings. These are probably the most significant differences between adult and children's hospice services.

The average number of admissions in one year will vary depending on the size of the hospice and the population served but is somewhere in the region of 391. The length of stay likewise is dependent upon the reason for admission and may vary from hospice to hospice but on average is between three and five nights.

Children's conditions

Children's hospices care for children and young people with a wide range of conditions. In general, less than 11 per cent of them have cancer. The conditions tend to fall into several categories as defined by ACT and RCPCH[2]:

'Group 1 – Life-threatening conditions for which curative treatment may be feasible, but can fail. Examples: cancer, irreversible organ failures of heart, liver, kidney.

Group 2 – Conditions where there may be long periods of intensive treatment aimed at prolonging life and allowing participation in normal childhood activities, but premature death is still possible. Examples: cystic fibrosis, muscular dystrophy.

Group 3 – Progressive conditions without curative treatment options, where treatment is exclusively palliative and may commonly extend over many years. Examples: Batten's disease, mucopolysaccharidosis.

Group 4 – Conditions with severe neurological disability, which may cause weakness and susceptibility to health complications, and may deteriorate unpredictably, but are not usually considered progressive. Examples: severe multiple disabilities, such as following brain or spinal cord injuries, including some children with cerebral palsy.'

The environment of a children's hospice

Although the philosophy of children's hospices is very similar to that of an adult unit, the environment is very different. Children are seldom to be found in bed. Even when very ill, they may spend much of the day in the main social areas surrounded by other children and the hustle and bustle of the hospice. Because it is important for the atmosphere to be that of 'home from home', there is little structure to the day, with care patterns following those of the child whilst at home. Staff, generally, do not wear uniforms and it can be hard to distinguish staff from parents or volunteers.

For a parent to decide to use a children's hospice is a very significant step and means that they must come to terms with the inevitability that one day their child will die. The initial visit can be a very difficult experience and many parents are reassured by the warm and friendly atmosphere which they encounter. They are often surprised on their first visit to be met with siblings running about and young people in electric wheelchairs moving at high speed and the hospice filled with noise and laughter.

There are however profoundly sad times when deaths occur. Children, although suffering from a continually deteriorating condition, may die quite suddenly and unexpectedly of an acute problem such as an infection. Not all deaths happen in the hospice, but even if the child dies in hospital or at home, it is possible for both the child and the family to come to the hospice to stay whilst funeral arrangements are made.

The number of beds varies from hospice to hospice. Some have as few as four whilst others as many as ten. The average number of beds of a children's hospice in the United Kingdom is approximately eight.

Reasons for admission

Children's palliative care needs differ, and there may be a variety of reasons for the admission of a child and some of these may include:

- Symptom control
- Deterioration of the child/young person's condition
- Support for carers to adjust to a new treatment regime
- Child entering the terminal stage of the illness
- Respite admission to give family a break
- A family crisis affecting ability to care for the affected child

Why involve volunteers?

Why, therefore, should volunteers be involved in a children's hospice? Although the tradition of volunteering in children's hospices is not as strong as in the adult sector, this had developed significantly during the last 5 or 6 years. Volunteers have a great deal to offer the many aspects of a children's service.

Firstly, they form strong links between the communities where they live and the hospice itself, helping to raise awareness, break down barriers, and increase understanding of the work of children's hospices. There is still ignorance and misconception about such work, and volunteers have a valuable role to play in dispelling myths. They bring a wide diversity of skills and life experience, which enhances that of the paid staff, allowing the hospice to offer so much more to the children and families for whom it cares. Volunteers are not so deeply involved with the problems of the families and bring with them a fresh approach and a new dimension to the care provided. They are one of the hospices' greatest resources and are exemplary ambassadors for the work of the organization.

Volunteer roles

There are many areas that may benefit from the involvement of volunteers and the following list is only an indication of some of the roles available:

- Activities with affected children and siblings.
- Befriending services for children, young people, and parents.

- Bereavement befriending.
- Complementary therapy services to children, families, and as staff support.
- Babysitting for siblings to allow parents to enjoy and evening out.
- Hydrotherapy pool aides.
- Driving—bringing families in to stay in the hospice or taking them out during their visit.
- Hairdressing and beauty therapy.
- Helping staff to prepare and serve meals.
- Helping with reception.
- Assisting with typing, filing, and photocopying.
- Housekeeping.
- Gardening.
- Assisting with general maintenance.
- Fund-raising: friends groups, servicing collecting cans, and helping with events.
- Public speaking—specially trained volunteers giving talks to groups about the work of the hospice.

Good practice recommends that volunteers should not be involved in any aspects of hands on clinical work nor should they be asked to undertake any unpleasant jobs that staff would not carry out themselves.

Planning for volunteer involvement

At the outset, it is important to make a strategic decision to involve volunteers, being clear as to the reasons as previously discussed in Chapter 3. The first step should be to develop a policy outlining the hospice's philosophy of volunteering and approach to their involvement. It is important to be clear about what volunteers will be expected to do or not to do and to appoint a Voluntary Service Manager to be responsible for recruitment and selection, induction, training, support, rostering, review, and management and smooth running of the volunteer programme.

To be truly representative, volunteers selected should reflect both the local and hospice communities in terms of age range, backgrounds, and ethnic origin. In children's hospices, a typical age range for volunteers is often between 16 and 75 and older.

Before recruitment takes place it is important to assess the types of roles which volunteers will be asked to undertake. Are they motivating, interesting, and varied? Role descriptions should be drawn up for each area of work, outlining the tasks to be undertaken, expectations, support, and supervision offered. This will clarify volunteer roles for staff and give volunteers a clear idea of expectations and boundaries.

Care must be taken, however, in the wording of all documentation relating to volunteers. Legal problems can ensue if volunteers can be deemed to have a contract and thus to be unpaid employees. This is discussed more fully in Chapter 8.

The recruitment process begins with the search for prospective volunteers. This continues through matching prospective volunteers' expectations with the needs of the hospice to allow volunteers to make an informed application. There are many different methods of recruiting volunteers outlined in Chapter 5, and the search for prospective volunteers is no different in the children's hospice environment.

It must be borne in mind throughout all stages of recruitment and selection, however, that working in a children's hospice environment is particularly challenging. Indeed Sister Francis Dominica[3] asserts that '..... in a society where we have come to see longevity as our right, the death of a child is experienced as outrageous.' Working in an environment where children die, therefore, can be at times an extremely emotional experience. It is not the best place for vulnerable people or for those who have recently experienced the death of a loved one, especially the loss of a child. Working with children also requires complete flexibility and the ability to be prepared to change plans to meet the needs and wishes of children.

Matching expectations and applications

Many prospective volunteers, however, have misconceptions about the work of children's hospices and, as a consequence, those making enquiries may have unrealistic ideas about the voluntary work they may be able to undertake. A significant number of people come forward wishing to read stories or play with the children. Whilst there may be opportunities for volunteers to be involved in these activities, it is more likely that the hospice really needs help in other very practical ways. It is important, therefore, to take time with would-be volunteers to match their expectations with the needs of the hospice and allow potential volunteers to self select at this stage. Such information sessions can be given either after the initial enquiry or after receipt of a completed application form.

Experience suggests that time taken at this stage of the recruitment process is time well spent and experience has shown that this results in high retention rates.

Recruitment and selection in children's hospices

The selection of volunteers is discussed in detail in Chapter 5, and this section highlights issues specific to volunteer management practice in children's hospices.

Once completed application forms are received, the process of matching skills with vacant volunteer roles can begin before inviting volunteers for interview to further explore their suitability. Particularly in children's hospices, volunteers should always be recruited for specific tasks. It causes ambiguity both for volunteers and for staff if volunteers are first recruited and then found 'something to do'. When this situation arises, often the volunteer does not know what they have come to the hospice to do and staff do not know what to ask them to do. The outcome of this is a frustrated volunteer who leaves and a member of staff who then believes that volunteers are at best ineffective and unreliable. Families may also be left confused as to the role of volunteers.

Key qualities of a volunteer in a children's hospice are the abilities to be completely flexible and to respond to the changing needs of the children and families.

Sometimes, those who have been used to a very structured working environment find adapting to the informal atmosphere difficult.

It is vital in any hospice that appropriate volunteers are selected for each role in terms of temperament, skills, motivation, or ability to undertake the required role. In a children's hospice, it is especially important to explore carefully with prospective volunteers their motivation for volunteering to work with children, attitude to children, and experience of young people whether in a paid, voluntary, or family capacity.

Especially important in selecting people to work with children is to build up a detailed picture of the prospective volunteer, and to make the right match of personality, skills, and experience (or ability to learn the skills) and to make a good match between the person and the role. It is also important to identify any person who is clearly unsuitable.

The interview

The importance of the interview has been previously highlighted in Chapter 5. Best practice in children's hospices recommends that interviews should involve the Voluntary Services Manager and another member of staff. This should be someone who will be supervising or working with the volunteer, as it is important to ensure that they have the opportunity to assess whether the prospective volunteer has the necessary skills and temperament for their area of work. It is important to keep interviews informal, friendly, and consistent. At the interview the following areas should be explored:

- Motivation/s for volunteering with a children's hospice.
- Their interest in, attitudes to, and experience of children.
- Experience of loss and bereavement, particularly relating to children.
- Exploration of how they feel they might cope when faced with the loss of a child they have come to know well.
- Expectations of voluntary work.
- Hobbies and interests.
- Health.
- Times available for voluntary work.
- Preference for type of volunteer role e.g. office or befriending.

The interview also gives an opportunity for prospective volunteers to ask questions and gain a better insight into the children's hospice environment. It is good practice for volunteers wishing to work directly with children to undergo a second interview which focuses on their motivations for working with children and their attitudes and approach to children using scenarios. (See Appendix A).

As a final part of the recruitment and selection process, any person in the United Kingdom wishing to work with children or vulnerable adults in a paid of voluntary, requires to undergo either a standard or an enhanced disclosure check. This is dealt with in more detail in Chapter 8.

Selection criteria for children's hospice volunteers

It is important to be clear about the qualities required by prospective volunteers to work in a children's hospice and to be clear about what would cause someone to be unsuccessful in their application. These criteria include:

- Genuine interest in the hospice's work.
- Clear reasons/motivation for volunteering in a children's hospice.
  (e.g. a love for children, time to give, to develop confidence, to gain experience for work, to give something back, to make friends, being a few of the most common).
- People who like people, especially children, and can work as part of a team.
- Approachable, flexible people.
- An empathy for the work of the hospice.
- Tact and sensitivity.
- Clear commitment and reliability.
- Appropriate skills for the task/s or ability and willingness to learn these.
- A Disclosure check clear of any convictions that would disqualify from working with children.
- People who have not experienced a recent bereavement, most especially of a child, and who would have the ability to work around loss and bereavement.

Experience has shown that most applicants prove to be suitable and are likely to be accepted as volunteers. Generally, this is attributable to the fact that they have given a great deal of thought before making an application and, in the early stages of recruitment, have had the opportunity to develop a clearer understanding of the hospice and the role of volunteers. From time to time, however, it will be necessary to turn down a prospective volunteer. Some of the reasons for doing so might include:

- Interviewers being unsure of the motivation for working with children.
- Someone who had been convicted of an offence against a child.
- An inappropriate attitude to disability or to children.
- Refusal to undergo Disclosure check.
- An immature young person.
- A recent bereavement, or unresolved loss, especially loss of a child.

Bereavement

Often people who have been recently bereaved see working in a hospice as a way of helping themselves to resolve their loss. However, working in a situation of frequent loss and bereavement serves only to re-awaken experiences and cause further distress[4]. People struggling themselves with a bereavement are also less able to support families and children facing loss. Often, parents of children who have died in the hospice wish to volunteer to give something back and this must be carefully explored and covered by the hospice's policy on volunteering.

Introductory training and support

Volunteer induction, like staff induction, is a process rather than an event and ideally takes place over the first 3 months of a volunteer's involvement with the hospice. This section is intended to follow on from Chapter 6 in focussing on induction topics specific to children's hospices. These should include:

- Information about the hospice's organizational structure and philosophy
- What the hospice care means to a family
- Brief overview of children's conditions
- Child protection
- Volunteering guidelines, expectations, and boundaries
- Where and how to access support

It is beneficial to provide new volunteers with a 'buddy' or mentor who may be an experienced volunteer or member of staff. This helps with support and training during the early weeks of involvement.

The end of induction review is important to hear feedback from the volunteer on their experiences and to give feedback on their performance. If problems have been identified either by the volunteer or the hospice, it is important that they are resolved at this point rather than let more time go by. It may be that additional training or a change of role is all that is required to remedy the situation. On rare occasions, however, it may be clear that the hospice is not the right place for the volunteer and it may be necessary to end the relationship.

Support and supervision

Support for everyone who works in a children's hospice environment is vitally important in order to prevent 'burnout'. The work can be emotionally draining and volunteers are just as vulnerable as paid staff. Experience suggests that they may even be more vulnerable as their link with the hospice is more tenuous and their support networks less solid.

Volunteer support therefore is of prime importance from the moment a volunteer becomes involved within the hospice as discussed in Chapter 7. This is a collective responsibility involving all members of staff and volunteer colleagues on a day-to-day basis. Effective support enables the volunteer to give of his or her best and reduces the turnover of volunteers.

Support comes in many forms both informal and formal and is especially important when a death occurs in the hospice. A breakdown of a possible support strategy for volunteers in one children's hospice is outlined below:

1 *Informal support*
- Day-to-day contact and involvement with staff and fellow volunteers.
- Regular 'open door' interaction with Voluntary Services Manager.
- Informal meetings and opportunities for discussion and exchange of ideas.

2 *Formal support*

- Pairing of new volunteers with a more experienced 'buddy' or mentor.
- Preparation for their role and ongoing information about the hospice.
- Volunteer support and development meetings as part of an integrated general training programme.
- Specific skills training.
- Review for new volunteers at end of induction period.
- Supervision sessions (individual or in teams) for all volunteers.
- One-to-one supervision and group supervision for bereavement befrienders, befrienders, and volunteers involved with children.
- Ongoing informal review.
- Support meetings following deaths of children.
- Spiritual support from hospice chaplains.
- Counselling service.

The importance of volunteer retention

If an effective volunteer recruitment and selection process is coupled with good support and supervision, volunteer retention is likely to be high. It is important to both the families and to staff that there is not a constantly changing team of volunteers.

Many people come into the life of the affected child and his or her family either during frequent hospital visits or in the home. In the hospice they also meet different staff and volunteers; and consequently seeing the same faces and getting to know them, is extremely important.

Continuity is also important to staff who invest time in training volunteers to become effective in their area of work. If there is a high turnover of volunteers, staff are continually training new volunteers. This can result in staff feeling that volunteers are more of a drain on their time than a valuable support. A volunteer who comes in regularly over a long period of time becomes very skilled in their role and is a great resource to the hospice.

Regular monitoring and review also has a key role to play in retaining volunteers.

Dealing with difficult situations

If there is a spirit of trust and respect between people working together, the number of occasions when serious problems arise should be minimal. If they do, however, it is important that guidance exists on how to deal with the situation. Volunteers and staff should be aware of the procedure for dealing with difficulties.

There are usually a number of options[5] open to the Voluntary Services Manager in dealing with difficulties with volunteers. These include:

- Retraining
- Finding a different role

- Asking the volunteer to take a break for a short time
- Mentoring

Except in serious cases, these options should be explored before deciding to ask the volunteer to leave. It may be necessary in the last resort, however, to ask a volunteer to leave and this should be done sensitively and with honesty. Reasons which would prompt the dismissal of a volunteer include:

- Inappropriate behaviour towards children, young people, or families
- Continual breach of boundaries with families
- Continual breaching of guidelines
- Breakdown of working relationships
- Theft, fraud
- Alcohol or substance abuse whilst on duty

Training

Ongoing training is an important part of helping volunteers to maximize their skills and effectiveness as highlighted in Chapter 6. Training also continues to keep volunteers motivated and increasingly, hospices are expected to ensure that volunteers in certain areas of work undertake 'statutory' training e.g. food hygiene, moving, and handling.

For volunteers working with children, it is vital that they undertake a preparatory course in addition to the induction programme. Such training may cover:

- Child protection
- Children's conditions
- Importance of communication through play
- Communicating with children without speech
- Dilemmas in working with children and families
- Conversing with families
- Dealing with issues around bereavement

Challenges of volunteer involvement in children's hospices

Where children are involved, there is often anxiety around inclusion of volunteers, and concern is expressed from time to time there are risks associated with the involvement of volunteers in the children's hospice environment. If volunteers are effectively recruited, selected, inducted, supervised, and managed, there should be no more risks attached to volunteers than to paid staff.

Any problems that may be encountered are far outweighed by the benefits. Problems often occur not because people are volunteers, but because when any group of people work together difficulties may arise.

The key role for the Voluntary Services Manager, therefore, is to ensure robust recruitment, selection, and management procedures to ensure the minimization of risk.

Boundaries

The informality of the children's hospice setting can be ambiguous for volunteers in terms of boundaries and 'friendship' with families. Often children and families become known to staff and volunteers over many years and build up strong bonds and relationships. Families may perceive staff and volunteers as 'friends' or even extended family, and it becomes essential to reinforce the role of professional boundaries with both staff and volunteers. Guidance is not only important for new volunteers, especially young people, both written and through ongoing training are key to maintaining the correct balance of relationships within the hospice.

Wherever volunteers and staff work together, there is the potential for difficulty arising from lack of understanding of each other's roles. Volunteers offering a service such as complementary therapies can engender professional rivalry or resentment with paid staff. This blurred boundary situation needs careful and sensitive management.

Flexibility and communication

The complete flexibility of the children's hospice environment can be difficult for some volunteers who have a need to be busy with an organized work schedule. For these people, the area of work must be chosen very carefully and they are seldom successful in working with children. Volunteers need to be patient, adaptable, and willing to change plans at short notice.

It can be difficult for new volunteers to know how to interact with profoundly disabled children and those with limited ability to communicate. They may also be apprehensive initially in talking to families, most especially bereaved families, anxious that they will say something inadvertently to cause upset. Effective induction and training is important in to preparing volunteers. The ongoing support and guidance of staff, however, is vital in helping them to develop skills and confidence in these areas.

Young volunteers

Many of the adolescents and young adults who use children's hospice services lack the opportunity to socialize with their peers, especially able-bodied young people. Whilst young people who need hospice care may have life-limiting conditions, they have the same interests, needs, and aspirations as their peers. Yet at a time when their peers are becoming more independent, the deteriorating conditions of life limited young people result at this stage in their increasing dependence on others.

Senior school pupils and students aged between 16 and 25 have much to offer, therefore, as volunteers. They have similar interests, talk the same language, and can offer opportunities for companionship and socialization.

Children's hospices, however, are often reluctant to involve this age group as they fear that they would need a higher level of support given their closeness in age to some of the affected children. A recent study[6] demonstrated that these fears were unfounded. Children's hospices who involved young volunteers found that with effective selection, support, preparation, and training, young volunteers can be a real asset to a children's hospice. The young volunteers reported that although initially anxious, they quickly settle. They cited the relaxed and friendly environment and the support of an older volunteer as being important. Young hospice users found mutual benefit in spending time with people of their own age, giving them an opportunity to share common interests and experiences and a sense of normality.

Conclusion

The rewards from involving volunteers in children's hospices are significant. Their generosity of time and spirit is immense. They offer children and families another avenue for support and other ears to listen. Volunteers can be many things to many people: a young able-bodied companion for affected teenagers; a young 'friend' for siblings to interact with; a peer for mums and dads to relate to; an older parent figure to understand and support; an extra pair of hands to share the load with staff; an added source of laughter and fun and, most importantly, another member of the children's hospice family.

Appendix A

Children's Hospice Association Scotland

Interview: Volunteers working with children

1 What made you want to come forward to work with the children?

    1.b. What age groups do you prefer to work with ?

2 What experience of children either in work or home life do you have which you feel will be helpful to you as a volunteer in this setting?

3 Discuss type of activities in which volunteers will be involved. How do you feel about this?

    3.b. What would you do if you found yourself with a group of five 4- to 12-year-olds and the Activities Coordinators were off ill?

4 What rights do you feel children have?

5 Whilst you are working as a volunteer you find a child behaving in a way that you personally find unacceptable. How would you handle this?

6 Any questions?

Explain about preparation day
Trial period

Decisions with reasons:

Interviewers: _____   _____

Date: _____
       _____

References

1 Association for Children with life-Threatening Conditions or Terminal Conditions and their Families/Royal College of Paediatrics and Child Health. (1997). *A Guide to the Development of Children's Palliative Care Services.* ACT/RCPCH.

2 Association of Childrens' Hospices (ACH). *What is a Children's Hospice?* Bristol, ACH.

3 Dominica, F. (1991). In *The Death of a Child* (ed. Wilkinson T.). London, Julia MacRae Books.

4 Gold, E. (1997). The Role and Need of the Children's Hospice in the United Kingdom. *International Journal of Palliative Nursing* 3(5), 281–286.

5 McCurley, S. and Lynch, R. (1998). *Essential Volunteer Management* (2nd Edition). London, Directory of Social Change.

6 Scott, R. (2004). Volunteering for the Future. An Evaluation of the Effects on Young Volunteers of Working in Palliative Care. *International Journal of Volunteer Administration* 22(2), 21–25.

Recommended reading

Armstrong- Dailey, A. and Zarbock Goltzer, S. (1993). *Hospice Care for Children.* New York, Oxford University Press.

Chapter 13

Volunteers working in a comprehensive palliative care service in Australia

Rosemary Hanley

The experience on which this chapter is based was gained from initiating, developing, and managing a palliative care volunteer service in a public hospital (or 'medical centre' as it is now more commonly called) in Australia. It had an active volunteer service for 4 years before a palliative care service was started.

The author's previous experience includes many years of coordinating volunteers in other types of services before moving into palliative care.

What is a comprehensive palliative care service?

A comprehensive hospice/palliative care service is one with inpatient beds, a hospital palliative care team working in an acute hospital, and a community palliative care service or a close working association with one. Often, it also includes a day centre (sometimes termed a day hospice), both educational and research facilities, and usually a bereavement service.

The hospital on which this chapter is based is a public (government-run) one, which also has a university research area. The hospital facilities are divided into four sections, one of which is the cancer section where the volunteer service is based.

The palliative care team provides care/consultancy services to:

◆ Cancer wards.

◆ Cancer outpatients (ambulatory) visiting the hospital.

◆ Palliative care patients throughout the hospital, whether or not they have a malignant disease.

◆ Palliative care unit with 20 beds.

◆ Liaison with domiciliary/home-based palliative care services (now usually referred to as a community palliative cares service).

The palliative care service is based in the cancer section of the hospital but its staff provide care and advice throughout the whole hospital.

The palliative care service

The palliative care consultancy team consists of:

◆ The medical director of palliative care

◆ A nurse consultant coordinator of palliative care

◆ Medical officers

◆ Consultant palliative care nurses

◆ Social workers

◆ Pastoral carers

◆ Dietitians

◆ Physiotherapists

◆ Occupational therapists

◆ Manager of palliative care volunteer service (VSM)

◆ Palliative care volunteers

The other dimension of the service is the 20-bed palliative care unit, which has a designated nurse unit manager and its own palliative care nursing staff, the Voluntary Services Manager (VSM), and the palliative care volunteers. The VSM and her assistants have offices near the palliative care unit.

A comprehensive palliative care service, like any palliative care service, provides holistic care for patients with life-threatening, incurable illnesses, and for their families and friends. The nurse coordinator of palliative care and the palliative care nurses are consultant nurses for the whole hospital.

They visit the patients, advise the staff, especially about pain control, and arrange for the patients' discharge from the acute wards to the palliative care unit, to a nursing home, to their own home, or to some other place of residence. Part of this discharge is organized with palliative care staff from a community-based palliative care service who will visit the patient at home. The staff of the hospital palliative care service liaise regularly with the community palliative care staff about patients they have in common, the former having got to know them when they were inpatients and the latter when they came back into the community for continuing care.

This chapter is about volunteers in the hospital and its palliative care unit settings, but it should be noted that the community palliative care services also have volunteers who visit patients at home. The two groups of volunteers as with the staff complement one another.

Volunteers

Why have volunteers in a comprehensive palliative care setting?

In this hospital, it was decided to appoint a VSM to initiate a palliative care volunteer service because the palliative care and other staff felt that the patients needed more holistic care than they had time to give. They knew that someone taking time to just 'be there'; to spend time with the patients was an important part of the patients' care and well-being. Unfortunately, funding is never enough to cover all needs, so volunteers were looked at as a solution.

Which conditions govern the work of volunteers?

> **Key point:** It must be stressed that volunteers complement but never supplement the clinical management of other team members or members of staff (see later in this chapter).

Volunteers may never do anything that is part of any staff member's job description. The VSM must not ask a volunteer to do a task that would contravene this agreement with unions and staff. Volunteers are only allowed to work up to 16 hours per week in this hospital.

Although, as mentioned earlier, it was initially envisaged that volunteers would save precious hospital funds they do not do so directly but indirectly. They help to make the patient feel better cared for, thus making the hospital run more smoothly and effectively. Another reason that volunteers are welcome in a hospital and hospice setting is that they bring to the patient's bedside some of the outside world. The patients see nurses, doctors, and other professionals all day long and quite often feel vulnerable because he/she is the only person who is not a medical professional.

Volunteers are never paid a wage but may be reimbursed for out-of-pocket expenses (e.g. petrol money for driving a patient, or for further education or training). Volunteers may never give an opinion on anything medical.

How to describe a volunteer

The volunteer is someone who:

- Like the patient, is not a health-care professional.
- Is not in a uniform but in normal everyday clothes.
- Is a mother, father, sister, brother, husband or wife, just like the patient.
- Has time to listen.
- Is willing to just be there giving his/her undivided attention to the patient.
- Can do little tasks for him/her.
- Can listen to the patient's worries or who will talk about anything but illness if that is what the patient chooses.
- Will take the patient for a walk even in a wheelchair.
- Will help with meals.
- Will help with grooming.
- Always respects confidentiality. In other words, a palliative care volunteer is a person who comes to see the patient with the specific intention of doing what the patient wants him/her to do within volunteer guidelines (see the Appendix). Palliative care volunteers are part of the interdisciplinary palliative care team and must act and expect to be treated with respect as are all members of the team, both paid and unpaid.

What do volunteers do?

Each working day, the volunteers come to their office, sign on, and read the patient notes written the previous day in the daily workbook. They then report for duty to the nurse unit manager (sister-in-charge) of the area in which they are working. Two volunteers work in each area, visiting patients separately from each other.

There are different times of duty and several different areas in which the palliative care volunteers work with the patients. They are:

- Day-roster
- Palliative care unit
- Radiotherapy
- Evening roster
- 'One-to-one' (1/1)
- Specialized work
- Office work
- Fund-raising

The aim is to have each volunteer on day-roster once a week, and in the palliative care unit once a week for about 4 to 6 hours each time. The volunteers prefer to keep to the same 2 days each week but are happy to go where needed at these times.

There are many different volunteers working in our hospital (e.g. fund-raising, canteen, drivers, in the accident and emergency unit) and in some of the other wards as well as the palliative care unit. Each group of volunteers must attend a specialized education programme before working in the hospital.

The VSM always has the final say on what the palliative care volunteer is permitted to do.

Recruitment of volunteers

A person who has had cancer or any debilitating disease needs to discuss it with the coordinator of volunteers (or VSM) when applying to become a palliative care volunteer. The general rule is 12 months free of illness after the last appointment with a doctor.

The 12-months rule also applies to a prospective volunteer who has had a close relative or friend die. Each individual situation needs to be looked at by the coordinator of volunteers and appropriate other staff members before a decision is made.

A volunteer needs to be physically and emotionally ready to work with people who are dying. There is no person with greater empathy for a patient than one with experience of illness, but only when that person is ready.

The palliative care volunteer is given a copy of the mission statement, policies, aims, procedures, guidelines (see the Appendix), and his/her job description at the beginning of the initial education programme.

A statement of commitment, promising to work for at least 12 months, is signed by the volunteer before beginning work in the hospital.

Areas where volunteers do not work

There are some areas of the palliative care service where volunteers are never engaged.

Included in these is when a patient has a 'nuclear hazard' sign on the door of his/her room. The volunteer then would not visit that patient for 48–72 hours after treatment, whilst radiation remains active. Another example is if a patient has a 'do not disturb' sign on his/her door, then the volunteer is asked to check with the nursing staff to see if this includes themselves. Often, this sign is only meant for visitors.

Volunteer work areas

Day-roster

On day-roster the volunteers work in the two wards and day-care oncology. They spend one day a week for a month in each place. It is important that the patients get to know the volunteers when in the acute care section of the hospital as this means they already feel comfortable when they subsequently meet them in the palliative care unit.

Haematology/oncology wards

If the volunteers are in the haematology/oncology wards or day-care oncology, they need to check which patients are 'palliative care patients'. They have priority but the volunteers also visit the other patients in these areas.

On each haematology/oncology ward the volunteers visit the patients offering to do anything they can for the patient within the volunteer guidelines (see the Appendix). Quite often, it is simply to have a talk to fill the patient's time. Sometimes, these talks can disclose information that needs to be passed on to a staff member. On such occasions, the volunteer will encourage the patient to speak to a specific staff member.

Volunteers also help with grooming and/or helping the patient to manage his/her food. The volunteer may encourage or help the patient to write his/her memoirs or read to the patient. If a patient is very unwell, the relative or friend who visits the patient regularly often appreciates the company of a volunteer.

Day oncology

In day oncology, where patients have chemotherapy or other day procedures, volunteers have a short chat with the patient and often with a family member or friend who is accompanying the patient. They make a cup of tea or coffee for the patients and distribute the lunches. There is a fairly rapid turnover of patients so the volunteers are kept busy.

Palliative care unit

Volunteers undertake similar work in both the cancer wards and the palliative care unit. Here, they spend more time sitting holding a patient's hand and helping with meals. They also take the patients out in a wheelchair around the hospital grounds. This brings the patient into contact with the world outside and gives him/her an opportunity to smell the flowers and feel the sun, etc. Volunteers also sit with dying patients if they have no family or friends present at this time.

Another volunteer occupation in this unit is spending time with patients' families either beside the patient's bed or in the lounge rooms. In this unit the volunteers take around the drinks trolley at lunch time.

Radiotherapy unit

Volunteers visit the radiotherapy waiting rooms and spend time waiting with the patients. This gives both the patient and their carer another chance to get to know the volunteers. It also gives the volunteer an opportunity perhaps to discover a patient's needs while the patient is still staying at home.

Evening roster

This is between 16:00 and 18:00 hours with two different volunteers on duty in each area.

The evening roster begins with a drink round where the volunteer takes a trolley of both soft drinks and alcohol to the patient's bedside or, if the patients are mobile, to a sitting room for pre-dinner drinks. (No alcohol is ever given to a visitor.) When this round is completed, the volunteer is then available to assist patients who need help with eating their meals.

The main point to emphasize is that volunteers help only when the patients cannot do things for themselves. Patients need to retain as much independence as possible.

This evening roster is usually a very pleasant, relaxed time for both volunteers and patients. Often, volunteers who cannot help during the day because of other commitments are able to help at this time.

'One-to-one'

A volunteer who works with a particular patient on a regular basis is called a 'one-to-one' or '1/1' volunteer. This really symbolizes how a 1/1 volunteer stands beside a patient with a connecting link between them.

Such 1/1 volunteers are usually allocated to patients with extra needs such as the following:

1 From the country, some distance from the hospital.

2 With very few or even no visitors.

3 Who are going to be in the hospital a long time.

4 Who need extra emotional support.

5 Whose relatives or friends doing most of the caring need extra support. This 1/1 volunteer will visit this particular patient regularly, perhaps two or three times a week while in hospital and will take a special interest in this patient each time he/she comes to the hospital either for outpatient, radiotherapy, or day-oncology visits. The patient/volunteer 'match' must always be kept in mind when selecting a 1/1 volunteer. The patient always has the right to refuse a visit from a volunteer. Volunteers are selected for this volunteer role according to the needs of the patients. This means that volunteers, even if they are able to do so, may not always have a 1/1 patient.

It is hoped that one day there will be sufficient volunteers to be able to assign each patient a 1/1 volunteer when they are given palliative care status.

Special work

Many volunteers have special talents, which they bring to the hospital, such as painting, meditation, massage, hairdressing or craft, etc. If it is appropriate and in accordance with the hospital's policy, such volunteers are invited to use these talents for groups or individual patients. Other volunteers may have valuable previous experience (e.g. in fund-raising) in which case they would be placed in that department (see following paragraphs).

Office work

There are volunteers who, for many different reasons, prefer to work in the office rather than with the patients; so they are trained to organize the rosters, write the newsletter, keep the statistics up-to-date, and many other ongoing tasks.

Fund-raising

The fund-raising team has one or two fund-raising efforts each year. This money is used to buy drinks for the drink trolleys, for volunteer education, and further training courses, as well as to buy specific items of equipment for the palliative care service such as an oxygen concentrator.

There is a fund-raising and volunteers' office in our hospital and this department's manager is the person responsible for both fund-raising and volunteer services. There is also a manager of volunteers in this office who is responsible for all other managers of volunteers in the hospital. The Palliative Care Voluntary Services Manager (PCVSM) registers the palliative care volunteers with this manager of volunteers. This department covers all volunteers for insurance.

This manager of volunteers must be notified, usually verbally, of any activities affecting the hospital or advertised outside the hospital, including fund-raising (e.g. when education programmes are scheduled and advertised).

◆ The fund-raising for the hospital is organized by a volunteer committee with many auxiliaries throughout the suburbs who work closely with the manager of the fund-raising and volunteers' office. There are other coordinators for volunteer driving of patients to appointments, the canteen and coffee shops, the accident and emergency volunteers, the volunteers in other wards. All coordinators of volunteers are under the umbrella of this central department but answer to our own departments first.

◆ In the palliative care volunteer service, the group of palliative care fund-raising volunteers would report to the PCVSM informally then report formally at the palliative care volunteers' monthly meeting where the decision to go ahead with a specific fund-raising venture would be decided. The palliative care volunteer service would then ask permission for this activity from the manager of the fund-raising and volunteers' office in a formal letter.

At the end of a roster

When volunteers are finished for the day they return to the office, fill in the report forms, write patient notes, and sign off before saying goodbye to the VSM. If the volunteer is going to be absent at any time he/she makes a note in the holiday book so that when the rosters are being prepared for the next month, these dates can be taken into consideration.

Regular ongoing training and education of volunteers

One of our aims, as VSM working in palliative care, should be to educate the volunteers to be professional palliative care volunteers.

Professional means '(a) having or showing the skill of a professional, competent; (b) worthy of a professional (professional conduct)'.[1]

In the palliative care volunteer service being described, there is an initial education programme followed by further educational opportunities to enhance skills and knowledge by such means as monthly meetings, training as mentors, the advanced palliative care workers education programme, and external education courses each year.

Initial pre-service training

It is very important to carefully select and train the palliative care volunteers before they begin working with the patients.

Experience shows that it is better to have fewer but good quality volunteers than more volunteers who, for one reason or another, turn out to be unsuitable.

Subjects covered in our 40 hour initial training programme include:

- ♦ Palliative care—philosophy and practise
- ♦ Confidentiality
- ♦ Rights and responsibilities of volunteers
- ♦ Rights and responsibilities of patients
- ♦ Spirituality
- ♦ Ethical issues
- ♦ Culture and religion
- ♦ Sexuality and illness
- ♦ The vulnerability of being a patient
- ♦ Death, grief and loss

The volunteer also needs to know and be comfortable with him/herself before he/she can be comfortable with a patient who is dying.

The most important part of the programme is communication and, therefore, 20 hours of the programme are devoted to this subject. It is essential for a volunteer to be able to listen and to communicate extremely well with a patient.

Occupational therapy, physiotherapy, and diet in palliative care are discussed by the palliative care team with the student volunteers. Radiotherapy and chemotherapy are also mentioned.

When the volunteers finish the programme they are again interviewed. If they are suitable, they then begin working in the hospital with a mentor.

Monthly in-service training

There are regular monthly meetings for volunteers with 1 hour allocated to education and 1 hour for debriefing and general discussion. Prior to the meeting, a newsletter including minutes of the previous meeting and rosters for the next month are sent to each volunteer.

The volunteers share lunch before this meeting. A speaker is invited to address a list of queries about palliative care, which volunteers prepared at the beginning of the year.

If there is a patient with an illness or a specific problem that the volunteers need more education about, then the VSM would ask the appropriate staff member to speak instead of someone from the list of speakers.

External education

The volunteers are encouraged to attend palliative care or volunteer education programmes offered by other organizations. The costs of attending these are often subsidized by the service.

Advanced education for palliative care workers

It was found that the volunteers had many questions and wanted more education after they had been working with patients for a few months. A survey was conducted asking what information and further training were wanted. This resulted in the 20 hour advanced palliative care workers' education programme being offered each year. To qualify for the programme, participants must have worked in palliative care for at least 6 months before undertaking this study.

In the 20 hour advanced training programme we take time to go more deeply into subjects such as:

- Radiotherapy
- Chemotherapy
- The cell cycle and cancer
- Grief
- Bereavement
- Complementary therapies
- Cancer research
- Dying in a palliative care unit
- Dying at home
- Other subjects to help the volunteers' understanding of palliative care in the home and in hospital

The assessments after each course have shown that the programme is well received by both palliative care and pastoral care volunteers working in palliative care from around the state.

Mentors

A 'mentor' is a person who has been a palliative care volunteer for at least 12 months and is considered suitable to mentor or guide another volunteer. Not all volunteers wish to be a mentor and certainly being a good volunteer him/herself does not necessarily make him/her a good mentor. These volunteers then participate in a 4 to 6 hour mentor training course, which includes how to:

◆ Communicate by discussing or offering suggestions in a positive way.

◆ Support and encourage the new volunteer.

◆ Report to the VSM verbally (informally) and written (formally) on the progress of the new volunteer.

◆ Show new volunteers where to locate people and places.

◆ Help the new volunteer to fill in forms, and deal with documentation.

The role of the VSM in the debriefing of volunteers

There are several opportunities for debriefing:

1 When a patient dies there is a debriefing of staff on the ward, and volunteers are encouraged to go to these sessions, which are usually organized by the nurse unit manager (sister in charge of the ward) or a palliative care staff member.

2 At the volunteers' monthly meetings we also talk about the patients' deaths and any issues that the volunteers raise.

3 Once or twice a year, or when there is a need, someone is asked to come in and debrief the group or speak about looking after oneself.

4 It is also very important for the VSM to formally debrief on a regular basis as well as having someone for the volunteer to talk to at any time.

5 If a volunteer has been a 1/1 with a patient who dies or has been particularly close to a patient in the unit, I always notify them of that patient's death and chat to them about how they feel.

6 If it is felt anyone needs a special debriefing then that will be carried out. Either the VSM will debrief the volunteer or, if more appropriate, will get one of the staff, such as the social worker or the pastoral care person from the palliative care service, to meet with him/her.

Burnout

It is important to be conscious of the possibility of volunteer burnout. This is why it is so important for the VSM to be readily available to drop everything and spend time with the volunteer if that is needed.

My policy has been to have an open door and I find this works much better than having only specific report/debriefing times. By this I mean that I encourage the volunteers to greet me when they arrive and to again call by my office as they leave. During this time we usually chat about how their day went in a very informal way, and

I can usually pick up if there is something that is worrying them or that they feel needs to be looked into for a patient. Then, if necessary, we talk more seriously about this either then or at an appointed time. Sometimes, it is something I have to take up with someone else, and then I let the volunteer know the results of the follow-up.

If a volunteer seems to be tired all the time or irritable or just seems uninterested in everything, this could be a sign he/she is exhausted mentally or physically. I discuss with the volunteer if it is to do with his/her work with palliative care or if it is from something going on in his/her life outside the hospital.

If it is something that is more serious or is something from his/her life outside we sometimes agree that it would be wise for the volunteer to have some time off. We set a specific length to this time (e.g. 2 weeks, 3 months), or what seems appropriate, then review this at a later date. During this time off duty I maintain contact with the volunteer by telephone.

Another option is to have the volunteers work for a short time in the office or elsewhere where there is no patient contact.

Many volunteers need to move on after a few years working in palliative care either because they need a change or because of changed circumstances in their life. It is important to recognize and to acknowledge the work they have done for the patients and the palliative care service.

Burnout is something that the VSM must watch for in him/herself. It is helpful to make a list of your favourite things that you can use to help relax you on a regular basis. Time away from one's regular routine is also beneficial.

Delegating responsibility

The primary duty of the VSM is to 'be there' for the volunteers, to be readily available. By delegating tasks this allows the VSM to be available rather than getting bogged down in routine office work.

Organizing and ordering supplies is one task that can be delegated as can setting up rooms for meetings, minute-taking, and writing reports on meetings. The formation of a volunteer fund-raising committee could also be delegated.

When it is planned to delegate responsibility to someone or to start something new, it is always discussed at the regular meetings of volunteers, clear plans drawn up, and a 'job description' prepared for whoever is asked to take on the responsibility. Reports from the person taking on the role are then presented at the regular volunteer meetings.

It is important that the VSM always knows what is going on by showing an interest without seeming to check-up or override the volunteers' decisions. Regular written reports from the delegated volunteers are important. Duties should be interesting and fulfilling to the delegated volunteer.

Accountability of the VSM

In the hospital on which this chapter has been based, the VSM answers to the nurse consultant coordinator of palliative care services first, but also to the manager of volunteers for the whole hospital.

Selecting volunteers for specific work

Volunteers who look after the specific parts of the programme are those who:

◆ Have a special interest in that area.

◆ Have already shown a talent in that specific.

These people have offered themselves as volunteers knowing they had a particular skill or experience that might be useful. Most volunteers come having heard of the work 'by word of mouth' but a few respond to advertisements. In that case, whatever special qualities they may have are discussed with them. They are asked if they have had the experience of having someone close to them die. It is possible from an initial informal chat that enough information is provided to decide whether to give them an application form or to advise them against applying. The application form asks among other things for special qualities, gifts or skills. If these skills are appropriate, the prospective volunteers are asked if they would be willing to use their talent with the patients. (We do not have children under the age of 16 in the cancer wards because they go to the children's hospital.)

Sometimes, volunteers are voted in at a meeting while at other times I personally invite them to undertake a task. Asking people to take responsibility for something that they are good at is a way of showing that what they do is noticed and appreciated.

It is very important to thank volunteers for what they do for the patients, the staff, and especially for helping the VSM.

When problems arise

If, on the other hand, a problem arises with a volunteer, the VSM will need to discuss the issue with him/her as soon as possible. It is always important to be honest with a volunteer but discuss the problem gently with him/her rather than say 'you are wrong'.

Quite often you will find that they too are not happy with what is going on but do not know what to do to change things. An open discussion allowing the volunteer to express his/her feelings, then working on the problem together and, if possible, getting them to find a solution makes things easier for everyone. In fact, this usually strengthens the volunteer's commitment to the palliative care service and to yourself as his/her VSM.

It is important for a volunteer to know that you respect his/her confidentiality just as you expect him/her to respect the confidentiality of patients and staff.

If the problem is between two volunteers, the VSM usually talks to them separately; then if they cannot solve the problem themselves, the VSM meets with them together and oversees the discussion. Sometimes, the circumstances are too raw and another action has to be taken (perhaps by transferring one or both to another duty). If it is not a major problem affecting the hospital or patients then it is sometimes better to let things rest for a while before instigating a meeting. This gives them time to cool down and think things through.

Key point: Remember, the patient's comfort is of the utmost importance.

When having a discussion with the volunteers about a problem I bring questions like these into the conversation:

- 'Why are you here?'
- 'Who have you come here to help?'
- 'Is this situation helping either the patient or you?'
- 'Is this too stressful for you or are you bringing your personal life into your voluntary work?'
- 'Do you need time off?'

For *major* problems with both staff and volunteers, there is a laid-down hospital procedure. If a volunteer has to be asked to leave it can usually be done by discussion and mutual agreement.

Aiming for a more comprehensive palliative care service

What could make a good palliative care volunteer service an even better one? What follow are my personal views, based on many years experience.

1 The structures to set up and run extra programmes take time that is not available with only a part-time VSM; therefore a *full-time VSM and a part-time assistant* would be an asset. This would allow the VSM more time for specialized volunteer training therefore preparing the volunteers to do more for the patients.

2 It is important for the volunteers to be able to speak to someone whenever they need to. If the VSM is not available, then someone, preferably the assistant VSM, or another nominated member of the palliative care team should be available.

3 To be able to give each patient a 1/1 volunteer as soon as his/her diagnosis is palliative would be ideal. This volunteer can be there for them through all his/her visits to the hospital—this would necessitate many more volunteers.

4 Three shifts a day on all cancer wards, especially the palliative care unit, are desirable. A morning roster from say 07:00 to 09:00 hours would enable volunteers to help patients with their self-care if need be and also with breakfast while the nurses are at the busiest time of their shift. If patients can have their personal care (shave, hair set, nails clipped and painted, etc.) completed early in the day, it helps them to face another day more confidently.

The volunteer only does what the patient needs and wants. This leaves the patient with as much independence as possible, for example, the patient may be able to shave himself quite well but cannot reach the razor in the drawer. Note: volunteers should never overwhelm patients.

The relationship between volunteers and staff

There is an agreement between the union and the manager of all the hospital volunteers as to how many hours a volunteer may work in a week. It is important to ensure that no volunteer works more than this number of hours or you will jeopardize the programme. In this hospital, this agreement is for 16 hours per week per volunteer.

Another important policy of the hospital is that volunteers may not do any of the work of paid staff. That is to say, they complement but never replace paid staff. This applies even when a health-care professional offers his/her services as a volunteer. If they are placed in a clinical environment they report to whoever is in charge of that unit of the hospital but do not replace any salaried member of staff. Never having had a doctor volunteer it is not possible to say what would be the case there.

It is wise for the manager of palliative care volunteers to regularly speak to staff individually or in groups about the volunteers' work.

Annual review

There is an annual review of each palliative care volunteer, which includes a written questionnaire and an interview. At this interview we set the aims the volunteer has for the next 12 months as a palliative care volunteer as well as discussing the questionnaire and any other issues. Even though these interviews take many hours I find that they are well worth the time spent.

Conclusion

The coordinator (as we still call her) or VSM, must always consider him/herself first—remembering that he/she is not there to solve all the problems of the patients or volunteers. It is vitally important to ensure that there is someone who has time to debrief the VSM regularly and that the VSM has other interests in order to relax.

Regular meetings with the multidisciplinary palliative care service in the hospital are essential as these meetings keep the professional palliative care team up to date with what is happening in the volunteer team, and the volunteer team with what is happening in the hospital. It is the responsibility of the VSM to update the team on volunteer activities.

It raises the profile of the volunteer team if the VSM takes a volunteer on a rotating basis to such meetings, discussing ideas in advance with the volunteer to save embarrassment.

Regular, even frequent, meetings with other coordinators of palliative care volunteers/VSMs in the city or district, can be very useful—sharing information and ideas, collaborating in education and training courses, being mutually supportive. It can be so helpful and reassuring to find that many problems and challenges are common to them all.

Appendix

Austin & Repatriation Medical Service, Palliative Care Volunteer Service Guidelines for volunteers*

1 Three months after a volunteer accepts his/her first patient or begins on the wards, there shall be a confidential review with the coordinator of the volunteer's role, thereafter an annual review will occur.

2 Observe confidentiality of patient, staff, and volunteers at all times.

3 In an emergency situation, call the nurse immediately.

4 Don't comment on a patient's treatment or medical condition.

5 Don't offer advice regarding a patient's personal or family matters. Generally, you can best help the patient or caregiver by letting them talk about their problems and by being a good listener.

6 Respect the right to privacy of patients and their relations.

7 Leave your own attitudes, values, and problems behind when you visit patients and their families. Treat the patient and family with the respect they deserve as fellow human beings.

8 Recognize and refer when a problem is beyond your abilities or your volunteer role. Inform the Coordinator of Volunteers or other Palliative Care Staff when problem situations arise or when professional or specialist intervention should be sought.

9 It is important that you care for yourself. There are times when your own emotional needs may have to come first. Don't be afraid to say 'No' if you are uncomfortable with a person or a situation. Try not to take problems away with you and recognize your own limitations.

10 Don't comment to patients on other patients or staff members.

11 Money and gifts are not to be accepted by volunteers. If a patient or relative wishes to make a personal gift, advise them that donations may be made to the Palliative Care Volunteer Service.

12 Do NOT give out your telephone number or address. Patients and caregivers can contact you through the Coordinator of Palliative Care Volunteers.

13 While how you dress may not matter to some patients, that may not always be the case. Be neat and appropriately dressed when visiting patients and their families.

14 A written report is required at the end of each day's activities.

15 Report regularly to the Coordinator of Palliative Care Volunteers. This will provide the support you need and keep the team informed so that the patient receives optimal care.

* Reproduced with permission from the Austin & Repatriation Medical Service, Melbourne, Victoria, Australia.

Reference

1 Moore B (ed.). (1997). *The Australian Concise Oxford Dictionary of Current English*, (3rd edition). Australia, Melbourne, Oxford University Press.

Recommended reading

Jordan, L. and Hanley, R. (2001). *Guidelines for Volunteers*. Melbourne, Victoria, Australia, Palliative Care Volunteer Service, Austin & Repatriation Medical Centre.

Chapter 14

Volunteers working in a community palliative care service

Kathleen Defellippi and Mabuyi Mnguni

This chapter tells the story of the development of palliative care in one region in South Africa. The history of the project was one of importing a UK model in the 1980s. By the 1990s, however, hospices were finding resources stretched by the challenges of working in areas of enormous disadvantage in which life-threatening diseases were very common. The chapter looks at how volunteers work in what might be regarded by many in the developed world as unusual, even unique community palliative care service in South Africa.

South Coast Hospice, Kwazulu-Natal, South Africa

South Coast Hospice (SCH) is situated on the eastern seaboard of South Africa alongside the Indian Ocean on the southern coast of Kwazulu-Natal. It provides palliative care within the UGU South Health District* that extends over approximately 3385 sq.km and has its headquarters in the town of Port Shepstone, just over an hour's drive south of Durban. (See Fig. 14.1 and Fig. 14.2.)

The palliative care service was developed against a background of enormous disadvantage, for example, the unemployment in this impoverished area by the late 1990s was 70 per cent[1] and the prevalence of tuberculosis was already 116 per 100,000 in 1998, one of the highest incidences in the world[2]. A survey by Murchison Hospital, which serves the area indicated that 82 per cent of people with TB were also HIV positive. At that time it was further estimated[3] that in South Africa as a whole 4.7 million people had HIV/AIDS, again one of the highest rates in the world.

The people of the area served by South Coast Hospice and its community palliative care service had access to primary care clinics offering round-the-clock cost-free care. In addition there were small hospitals offering 24 hour care, with minimal charges for medications. The clinics and the hospitals were state-run and state-funded unlike the palliative care services.

General practitioners (GPs) were readily accessible in urban areas. Patients could choose which ones to consult but were charged fees, which usually included medications, but at a cost usually much higher than a hospital would charge.

---

* UGU is a Zulu word meaning 'the coast'.

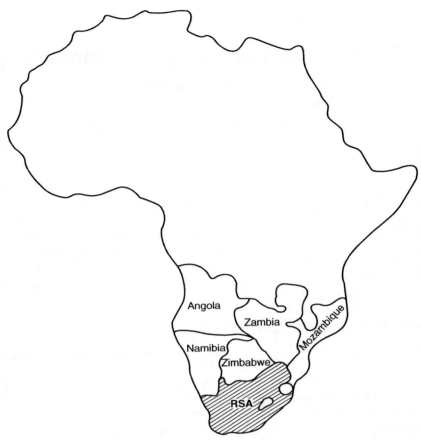

Fig. 14.1 The continent of Africa showing the Republic of South Africa (RSA).

The impact of HIV/AIDS

The magnitude of the HIV/AIDS problem in South Africa is enormous and the problems faced by the patients and carers are more than physical. The psychological effects and the stigma related to HIV vary as the infection progresses.

The response by the hospice to the HIV/AIDS problem had to deal with how people reacted to diagnosis. Typically, this followed a similar pattern to any diagnosis of life-threatening conditions: at the initial 'well-but-worried' and healthy carrier stage, adequate counselling was often not sought. The infected person came to terms with his/her diagnosis by going through a series of psychological reactions, shock, fear, denial, anger, blame, and guilt. These universal reactions seemed to be exacerbated in the case of a person living with HIV/AIDS (usually abbreviated to PWA). The high level of stigma and lack of acceptance of the PWA often meant that people were frightened or ashamed of having a PWA in their home. This was to make it difficult for a

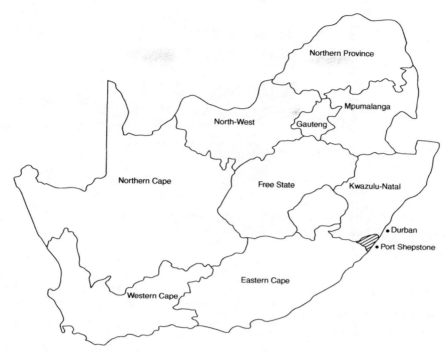

Fig. 14.2 Map of the Republic of South Africa showing the area (shaded) served by the South Coast Hospice.

volunteer/caregiver to have access at this time. It often took a while for these people to disclose their status to the family.

The bulk of the care the hospice was able to provide through volunteer involvement occurred when the PWA was already ill. As a result, the volunteer frequently had to deal not only with the terminally ill patient but also an overwhelmed family and the problem of stigma.

During the period described—the late 1990s, in excess of 60 per cent of PWAs referred to South Coast Hospice (SCH) were female. More than 80 per cent of all infected women acquired the HIV infection from a male partner to whom they had been faithful[5]. The skill level needed by volunteers to talk openly about sexuality and related health problems in a culture where such discussion is taboo and where 'Vulnerability to AIDS is often associated with a lack of respect for the rights of women and children'[6] was very great indeed. The project found that the problem was exacerbated when the volunteer was young and/or unmarried and had to deal with an older male who was culturally perceived as powerful. A relationship of trust was crucial for effective ongoing counselling and care to occur.

Figure 14.3 and Table 14.1 are taken from the UGU South HIV/AIDS/STD/TB Pilot Site Interim Report covering the period October 1999 to April 2001. This SCH research

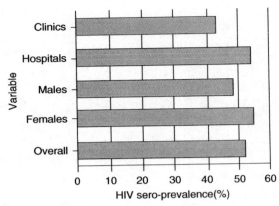

Fig. 14.3 HIV sero-prevalence of 12 000 clients tested at Port Shepstone Regional Hospital (Data collected September 1998–November 1999).

Table 14.1 Five main reasons given for a self-referral for HIV/AIDS (April 1998–May 2000)

Reason for self-referral	Number (%)
1 Interested after health education talk	1801 (73)
2 Client is ill	357 (14)
3 Client concerned about his/her risk activities	037 (12)
4 Client concerned about partner's risk activities	149 (6)
5 Partner is ill or has died	51 (2)

project demonstrated the magnitude of the impact of HIV/AIDS in the operational area of rural Kwazulu-Natal[7]. With no anti-retroviral medications available in South Africa at that time, it is daunting to think that the project faced the prospect of virtually *all* these HIV positive people requiring palliative care. Clearly, the project needed to find many dedicated volunteers if the problem was to be tackled.

The history of volunteer involvement

South Coast Hospice needed to develop innovative ways of coping with the overwhelming and escalating number of HIV positive people in their region in desperate need of holistic palliative care. How this was been done is the subject of the rest of this chapter.

SCH was working under severe financial constraints, support from the government accounted for just 6 per cent of the 2001 annual budget. All these factors resulted in SCH focussing on training *lay* community care-givers and volunteers to do work that is traditionally done by nurses and social workers. Professional nurses and social

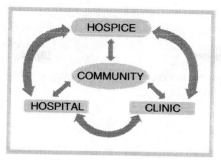

Fig. 14.4 Integrated community-based home care (ICHC).

workers were, in turn, required to concentrate on supporting and supervising these lay caregivers. The challenge of providing quality of care in this context was ever present.

As early as 1984, SCH found it necessary to adapt the British model and began collaborating with primary health-care clinics in order to provide holistic care to cancer patients living in the outlying rural areas. Many of the professional nurses who were working in outlying primary health-care clinics became hospice volunteers. But the scale of the issues that needed tackling meant that soon volunteers were not trained nurses but lay women eager to help people in their own district, usually within walking distance of their own home. Working in this way in their own community had the advantage that the volunteers were well known and relatively safe, although they were advised to work with a partner for additional support.

This rural outreach programme laid the foundation for the integrated community-based home care (ICHC) model that came about in 1996, in response to the escalating HIV/AIDS epidemic (see Fig. 14.4).

The following sections share the experiences of recruiting volunteers for community work in impoverished areas.

Definition of a volunteer

Volunteers form an integral and enriching part of hospices all over the world. To volunteer is to give service willingly of one's own accord. The biblical adage that in giving we receive, is true. The satisfaction that comes from making a positive difference in difficult circumstances is definitely rewarding.

In the developed world it goes without saying that no monetary payment is expected, or received, when one volunteers. However, this may not be the case when people from an impoverished background 'volunteer'. Their motivation may well be twofold. They genuinely wish to be of service and simultaneously hope that this 'volunteering' will lead to a job or gain them some incentive that will help alleviate their own plight by assisting them to feed themselves and their family. In view of this, the concept of a 'paid volunteer' is therefore not as strange as it may first seem. Hospices in Kwazulu-Natal grappled with sustainable ways of addressing this problem.

Volunteers did receive rewards, which ranged from food parcels to financial stipends equal to a nominal salary. The number of volunteers, their commitment, and the approximate number of hours they devoted to the hospice were some of the factors that needed to be considered. But as with any form of volunteer involvement, to prevent conflict, it is important to have a clear policy that is strictly adhered to and communicated to all concerned.

Selection of volunteers

The project realized that careful selection becomes even more important when payment of volunteers may be involved. It is therefore vital to ascertain the true motivation of any potential volunteer.

The universal qualities required for a person who will be working as a volunteer member of a team anywhere include:

◆ Personal warmth

◆ A non-judgemental attitude to those with HIV/AIDS

◆ Ability to communicate effectively

◆ Respectful and positive attitude to HIV status

◆ Flexibility and emotional maturity

◆ Well balanced lifestyle

◆ Good coping mechanisms

In South Africa *additional* characteristics found to be important include:

◆ A track record of community involvement

◆ The ability to communicate cross-culturally with sensitivity and respect

◆ The ability to converse in a knowledgeable and compassionate manner about HIV/ AIDS

Almost all volunteers are women because, traditionally and culturally, the women are the carers in this society. Caring is seen as one of their responsibilities.

Community-based volunteers seem to have a surprisingly low turnover rate. The most common reason for resignation is securing a better paid position. When this occurs, the hospice celebrates with them and they continue to be valuable ambassadors for the organization. Even when volunteers leave the geographical area they frequently volunteer for similar work in their new place of residence.

Introducing volunteers to the work

As important pillars in the provision of care it is necessary for volunteers, not only to be adequately trained for the work but also to be introduced to the key figures and all relevant role players in the community they will be serving. These include representatives from various government departments, non-governmental community-based organizations, and recognized community leaders. At the same time, the community needs to be informed about the programme as well as the role of the volunteer. Scheduled community meetings can often be used for this purpose.

It is also necessary to orientate all hospice professional staff regarding the training, skills, and areas of volunteer operation. In addition to making the volunteer feel a part of the organization, importantly, proper orientation also enhances the referral system.

New volunteers need to be given information about the correct channels of communication. They need to understand about supervision and relevant networking resources, in keeping with their specific job description. To avoid tensions building up between lay volunteers and hospice professionals, working relationships must be clearly defined from the outset. It is also important they be made aware of the need for flexibility. SCH volunteers rotated through the inpatient unit had to, of necessity, be prepared to work in a variety of areas. Experienced volunteers are often expected to shoulder additional responsibilities and mentor new recruits.

Relationship of volunteers to professionals

Whenever volunteers are involved in giving direct patient care, it is necessary to stress professional accountability. It is essential to have clear job descriptions that set out what is expected of the volunteer and also what he/she is not permitted to do.

As a general rule, non-professional volunteers and all lay caregivers do not liaise *directly* with professionals from other organizations. If volunteers encounter a problem when visiting a patient, they have access to registered nurses based at the primary health-care clinics scattered across the country. These nurses provide interim professional support until the problem can be reported to a palliative care nurse at the base palliative care unit/hospice. Should medical help be needed it is the palliative care *nurse*, not the volunteer, who brings the matter to the doctor's attention.

Volunteers may only administer medication according to a strict protocol. Generally speaking, they do not do so, but they are permitted to help a patient or relative to measure medicines. They do not carry out any invasive procedures.

The Hospice Association of South Africa (HASA) adopted and piloted the ICHC model (see Fig. 14.4) in which hospices work closely with various other HIV/AIDS community-based initiatives. The HIV/AIDS epidemic motivated numerous South African hospices to implement this practical model of care.

How integrated home-based home care operates

Developing how the hospice cared for PWA, included identifying patients at local hospitals who were then visited by South Coast Hospice community caregivers. The team transported patients home on discharge and informed the relevant primary health-care clinic. A full patient/family assessment was carried out and a care plan compiled on the first home visit.

Hospice care teams (salaried professional staff) visited on average once a week, interim support and care was provided by the trained lay volunteers who lived within walking distance of the patients' homes.

On average, each lay volunteer had about five patients and their families to visit. At the end of each week, each volunteer met with the Voluntary Service Manager (VSM) and the nurses and reported on the week's work.

In the event of problems developing between the weekly visits, volunteers and/or family members consulted with a professional nurse at the clinic who gave advice and medication if appropriate or, in the case of an emergency, arranged for admission to hospital. Hospice caregivers and volunteers networked with various other role players such as churches, women's groups, traditional healers, and other relevant individuals and groups, to obtain additional support for patients and their families. The core elements of the ICHC model (see also Fig. 14.4) included:

- Linking palliative home-based care to preventive care
- Providing a continuum of care
- Drawing on the strengths already existing in community-based care initiatives
- Integrating the statutory and private health-care sectors
- Training people from the community as caregivers and providing them with jobs
- Enhancing the morale of *all* health-care providers
- Capitalizing on important teaching opportunities

Involving volunteers to complement a small core of salaried community caregivers all care was audited on a 6-monthly basis, using an audit tool developed by the Hospice Association of South Africa (HASA) (see Appendices 1–3) during the piloting of the ICHC model. Although paid community caregivers were crucially important to the ICHC model, lay volunteers played a pivotal role in its success. The small core of paid caregivers could only manage to visit patients once a week, all others being done by the lay volunteers.

The work of volunteers

In South Coast Hospice, as in many hospices, the traditional roles for volunteers include:

- Direct patient and family care
- Fund-raising
- Administration
- Financial management and
- Numerous support and consultancy services

In keeping with the holistic care requirements of the developing world, hospices in Kwazulu-Natal also use volunteers for:

- Community development
- Poverty alleviation
- Orphan care
- HIV/AIDS awareness and prevention programmes

All this has become necessary because the traditional safety net provided by the extended family system in rural African communities is being eroded by HIV/AIDS[4]. In addition, there are the continuing social problems of poverty, unemployment, and domestic violence[4]. Overburdened grandmothers, who are themselves in need of bereavement support, cannot possibly cope with caring for their own sick children and grandchildren as well as inheriting the orphans. According to SCH statistics, 40 per cent of orphaned children are themselves HIV positive. This places an unimaginable burden on these elderly women, often themselves ill and frail and underfed.

Training

Ideally, volunteers should receive initial training:

* In their own geographical area.

* In an environment with which they are familiar.

* Preferably in their own language. Familiarizing them with community resources and how to access them forms part of this initial training. Training is based on the 3-month Hospice Association of South Africa (HASA) curriculum. When circumstances do not permit for the entire curriculum to be completed initially, core elements of each of the modules are incorporated into a 1-month course and the balance incorporated into ongoing/in-service training.

The curriculum is divided into the following eight modules and learning outcomes:

1 Introductory module—HIV/AIDS in context

On completion of this module, the volunteer must be able to demonstrate an understanding of the basic facts regarding the mode of transmission, prevention, and factors increasing the risk of the spread of HIV/AIDS and the role of home-based care.

2 The community caregiver

This includes an assessment by the student of his/her own values and attitudes to HIV/AIDS, as well as community misconceptions and myths. The role of the caregiver, rules of conduct, ethical principles, and professional approach, as well as support systems available to the caregiver.

3 Basic communication skills

On completion of this module, the volunteer is expected to be able to demonstrate effective communication skills and the use of interpersonal skills to establish rapport with patients and families, use correct referral procedures, keep accurate records, and have an awareness of ethical and legal issues.

4 Psychosocial and spiritual support

The social, emotional, and spiritual impact of the disease on the individual and family; the dying process; loss, grief, and bereavement, and how to offer support are covered in this module.

5 Basic nursing skills—including the philosophy of holistic care

Volunteers must be able to maintain basic hygiene and apply universal precautions in preventing the spread of infection, demonstrate a basic understanding of all the body systems, recognize specific problems related to HIV/AIDS, and be able to utilize this knowledge in the appropriate care of patients. They also need to be able to give sound nutritional guidance to patients and families.

6 Pain and symptom control

In terms of learning outcomes, the volunteer must be able to demonstrate an under-standing of total pain and its effect on the patient; identify non-pharmaceutical methods of pain relief and utilize simple appropriate measures for relieving pain. They must also work under professional supervision in the administration of pre-scribed medication. Students must be able to give an accurate report on all aspects of the patient's condition and employ proper storage and record keeping of medicines.

7 Paediatric AIDS

This module deals with all aspects of the disease and treatment related specifically to children. The volunteers are required to identify and respond to specific HIV/AIDS problems that relate to infants, children, and teenagers.

8 Teaching methods module

This is included so that community caregivers and volunteers are able to use relevant teaching methods to convey information to patients, families and communities, and use knowledge to empower their own communities in self-help.

Once the 3-month basic training is completed, volunteers are encouraged in identify-ing their own ongoing training needs. Volunteers bring with them a wide range of valuable experience that can often be appropriately channelled into peer training.

Support

Training forms an important part of volunteer support in that it affirms their compe-tency and contributes to their personal development and confidence. Community recognition of the sacrifice and committed dedication of volunteers is of paramount importance and certainly contributes to their sustainability.

Personal supervision and mentorship

Volunteers, particularly those working in impoverished and traumatic conditions need to be able to vent their feelings and talk about how the work is affecting them personally. Time needs to be scheduled for volunteers to have regular sessions with a suitably skilled psychosocial professional individually and/or in groups. In order to avoid 'burnout', volunteers are encouraged to set limits and work within a scheduled time frame. They are also encouraged to take time off on a regular basis.

Recognition

A badge or uniform means a great deal to hospice volunteers who are proud to be associated with the organization. Thanking volunteers encourages and motivates them, particularly when this is done in public. It makes profound sense to ensure that the contribution made by volunteers is stressed in all relevant reports. Everyone likes to be appreciated.

Volunteers associated with Kwazulu-Natal hospices together with their partners, are invited to attend two annual events—a 'Thanksgiving and Remembrance service' and a Christmas party.

Monitoring and evaluation

It is as important to monitor the quality of work done by volunteers as that done by salaried staff. With adequate preparation and a non-threatening approach, this can be perceived as uplifting and give volunteers a feeling of security. Regular assessment and feedback regarding the quality of their work is another way of telling volunteers that they are important.

Having a policy regarding the monitoring and evaluation of volunteers in place makes it easier to respond effectively to incidences of misconduct. For instance, the breaking of patient confidentiality is regarded as a dismissable offence. Evaluating the quality of work simultaneously monitors the effectiveness and relevance of existing training programmes. It also highlights areas that need to be included in ongoing training.

Enrichment

The following vignettes illustrate how the lives of just two people have been enriched by their voluntary involvement with the hospice. It is almost overwhelming to consider the vast number of hospice volunteers worldwide in terms of extrapolating the tremendous personal growth and inspiration that has benefited countless numbers of people. This staggering figure can be further multiplied by the numbers of patients, families, and friends who have, in turn, been able to experience an improved quality of life because of the generosity of hospice volunteers.

> I joined the hospice after working through a traumatic period in my own life. I felt that helping others would help me, which it certainly has done. I have gained knowledge through the very interesting training courses. Working with patients has taught me compassion, humility, and tolerance. As sick as they are, the patients and their families are very grateful for anything one does for them. Their gratitude is touching. I have learned that the few patients who are demanding just need to be listened to and understood. I admire the many dedicated people who work for hospice, both the staff and my fellow volunteers. Sometimes I wonder how the world would ever have managed without the Hospice Movement. (Pam)

> I have been a volunteer with South Coast Hospice since the early eighties and have developed experience and a wide knowledge in dealing with terminally ill patients. At first, most of the patients had cancer, particularly of the cervix or oesophagus, lately most of our patients have AIDS. I have gained a greater understanding of community and family dynamics. It is great to enjoy so much respect from the community, they really appreciate my services as a volunteer. Initially, my husband was not sure that my being a volunteer was a good idea, but all the positive feedback from the community has made him proud and very supportive of my work. In the beginning, I worked in the urban area but was able to be instrumental in getting hospice services to my own outlying rural area. (Nomangesi)

The value of volunteers

In addition to bringing so much 'heart' into a professional organization, the generosity of volunteers allows hospices to extend their service to reach vast numbers of people in need. Without volunteers, many of those in the greatest need might not be able to benefit from the sensitive, holistic palliative care, which hospices in the developing world strive to provide. In sub-Saharan Africa, volunteer care of HIV positive people also has important spin-offs for prevention relative to the rampant HIV/AIDS epidemic. By looking after HIV positive people, caregivers demonstrate to others in the community that there is no risk of becoming infected through everyday contact[8]. They also practise and teach universal precautions as appropriate.

Conclusion

The HIV/AIDS epidemic is presenting hospices in the developing world with enormous challenges and opportunities. Challenges, as these organizations become increasingly reliant on committed, quality volunteer input. Volunteers are a potential human resource which needs to be developed and nurtured. The challenges are accompanied by unprecedented opportunities in terms of the recognition of hospice expertise and credibility. How hospices respond to the escalating needs for palliative care will have a profound effect on individual organizations. It will also affect the future form and course of palliative care as well as its position in the formal health care sector[9]. The fact that government hospitals feel overwhelmed by the demands of the epidemic has undoubtedly contributed greatly to their collaboration with palliative care services, which is so necessary for the success of the integrated community-based home care model. Hospices in sub-Saharan Africa are currently in a strong position in terms of impacting on health-care policy. The Hospice Association of South Africa is actively lobbying for a quality palliative care component to be included in government home-based care programmes.

Appendix 1

The Hospice Association of South Africa (HASA) audit tool*
Palliative care audit instrument: client or family interview

Site:_____   Date:_____

Interviewee(s):_____

Choose a client who is bedridden or almost bedridden for this interview, but one who can speak and understand questions.

NR	ITEM	YES	NO
1	Where you given the opportunity to discuss your needs and problems?		
2	Did you feel that these were adequately addressed?		
3	Were you given sufficient information to enable you to understand and plan treatment and care?		
4	Was your pain controlled to your satisfaction?		
5	Were other symptoms controlled to your satisfaction?		
6	Did you receive support from other health professionals when you needed it to meet your needs? NB: this item is also N/A in areas with limited provider options		
7	Were you referred to other health services when necessary? NB: this item is also N/A in areas where service options are limited		
8	Have you received sufficient information and training from health-care workers to enable you to cope at home? NB: this item is addressed mainly to carers		
9	Do you know how and where to contact them (community caregivers) if you need assistance?		
10	Do you feel that the health-care workers have kept information concerning you and your condition confidential?		

Note: NA, not applicable. Use this when an item does not apply to the client, and explain why you do this. Not Asked, use this when you choose not to ask a specific question (e.g. you cannot ask item 10) if a family member who is not in the confidence of the client is present during the interview.

* Appendices 1–3 have been reproduced by kind permission of the Chief Executive of the Hospice Association of South Africa (HASA).

Appendix 2
Palliative care audit instrument: Palliative care units

Unit:_____ Date:_____ NR of beds:_____
On interview:_____

NR	ITEM	YES	NO
1	**Training**		
1.1	Is there a written record of In-Service Training?		
1.2	Do the records show that at least three levels of health-care workers have received in service training over the past 2 years?		
1.3	Are the following included in the In-Service Training Programmes?		
1.3.1	Holistic approach to pain management		
1.3.2	The WHO Pain Ladder		
1.3.3	Holistic approach to symptom control		
1.3.4	Psycho-social care of client and family		
1.3.5	Spiritual care of client and family		
1.3.6	Legal and ethical aspects		
1.3.7	Use of the referral system or network of care		
1.3.8	Bereavement care		
1.3.9	Family support		
1.3.10	Patient advocacy		
2	**Resources**		
2	Is there a list of resource organizations and persons including HIV/AIDS resources in the area to whom the client and family may be referred?		
2.2	Is there a named interdisciplinary resource team available for the primary care provider?		
2.3	Is there access to an identified ethics committee		
2.4	Are there documented methods to access grants and other forms of social assistance? NB: if a social worker is available to take care of these aspects, this is N/A		
2.5	Is there access to medication according to patient needs?		
2.6	Is there a referral form available for use?		
2.7	Are support groups and/or counselling services available for families and significant others?		
2.8	Is counselling available for clients about treatment options, prophylaxis, and other issues?		

3	**Policies and guidelines**			
3.1	Are there written policies on:			
3.1.1	Criteria for access to the care? NB: this refers specifically to which clients are assisted at which services; if these criteria are clear, this gives a YES			
3.1.2	Infection control?			
3.1.3	Treating health-care workers exposed to accidental infections (e.g. needlestick injuries)?			
3.1.4	Handling pain medication (ordering, storage, and administration)?			
3.2	Are the following guidelines or protocols available?			
3.2.1	Clinical			
3.2.2	Psycho-social			
3.3	Are guidelines reviewed annually?			
3.4	Holistic identification and support of AIDS orphans			
4	**The care team**			
4.1	Do members of the care team have access to:			
4.1.1	Structured support programmes in on-duty time? NB: a structured programme refers to regular and scheduled meetings or times			
4.1.2	Support in coping with illness, dying, and bereavement as needed; NB: this item refers to support when the staff needs it			
4.2	The unit has an adequate skills mix in the staff to cope with client care			
4.3	Staffing levels makes palliative care possible; NB: this refers specifically to going beyond physical care only			
4.4	Written job descriptions reflect a palliative care focus			
4.5	Suitably skilled supervisors to provide support; NB: this refers to a person with palliative care or mental health-care training			
4.6	Does communication in the team enhance care?			
4.7	Are updated treatment guidelines or protocols available to inform staff of recent policies?			
4.8	At least one member of the team is trained in palliative care			
4.9	Non-professional members form part of the team			

Record review

NB: Please choose 3 charts for every 10 beds in the unit. Exclude comatose patients.

NR	ITEM	YES	NO
5	**Do the records show that:**		
5.1	The client and family is the unit of care?		
5.2	The physical needs of the client and family have been identified?		
5.3	The psycho-social needs of the client and family have been identified?		
5.4	The spiritual needs of the client and family have been identified?		
5.5	Pain is managed holistically? NB: there needs to be evidence of interventions other than medication used for pain control for a YES		
5.6	Pain and other symptoms are managed to the client's satisfaction? NB: there needs to be evidence of patient reaction to nursing intervention showing improvement or satisfaction for a YES		
5.7	Symptom management is done holistically? NB: there needs to be evidence of interventions other than physical for a YES		
5.8	The WHO Pain Ladders are used in the management of pain? NB: there needs to be evidence of higher levels of pain control interventions being used in later stages of illness for a YES		
5.9	Each client has a named primary care provider?		
5.10	Therapeutic, psycho-social, and spiritual care resources have been mobilized when needed?		
5.11	Is there documentation to show that the client and family, when appropriate, received training in:		
5.11.1	• Self-care?		
5.11.2	• Use and side-effects of medication?		
5.12	Are the following charts included in the client record where applicable?		
5.12.1	Pain charts		
5.12.2	Medicine charts		

Appendix 3

Palliative care audit instrument for community services

Site:_____ Date:_____

Choose at least three client records of those who were not comatose for the main period of care.

NR	ITEM	YES	NO
1	Is there an adequate transport system to enable carers to reach clients?		
2	Is there sufficient equipment for loan/hire for clients?		
3	Are there back-up beds in the community for admissions?		
4	There is a policy or system for follow-up of clients who do not comply with referrals?		
5	In the case of client-held records, is continuity of care recorded?		
6	Do records show that clients have been assisted to continue involvement in life to the limit of his/her capacity?		
7	Is there documentation to show that the client and family receive training in:		
7.1	Self-care?		
7.2	Use and side effects of medication?		
7.3	Home medicine charts?		
8	Is home charting of medicines accurate?		
9	Supervision		
9.1	Formal supervision of community caregivers is done		
9.2	There is evidence of home visits by professional supervisors		

References

1 Health Systems Trust (HST). (1998). *HST Update*. Pretoria, HST, South African National Department of Health.

2 Strachan, K., South African Department of Health (SADH). (1998). *SADH Report*. Pretoria, South African National Department of Health.

3 Murchison Hospital. (1999). Unpublished report. (Available from Murchison Hospital, Port Shepstone, South Coast, Kwazulu-Natal, South Africa).

4 Hunter, S. (2000). *Reshaping Societies: HIV/AIDS and Social Change*, p. 129. New York, Hudson Run Press.

5 UNAIDS Point of View. (1997). *Women and AIDS*, p. 2. Geneva, UNAIDS.

6 UNAIDS. (2000). *Report on the Global HIV/AIDS Epidemic*, p. 37. Geneva, UNAIDS.

7 Campbell, L. (2001). *Interim Report UGU South HIV/AIDS/STD/TB Pilot Site*. (Unpublished).

8 UNAIDS. (2000). *Report on the Global HIV/AIDS Epidemic*, p. 87. Geneva, UNAIDS.

9 Defilippi, K. M. (2000). Palliative care issues in sub-Saharan Africa. *International Journal of Palliative Nursing*, 6(3), 108.

Chapter 15

Volunteers working in a tertiary referral teaching hospital

Suzanne O'Brien and Ellen Wallace

The role of a volunteer working within a tertiary referral hospital palliative care service in Canada, although similar in many ways to that of someone working in a free-standing, privately funded or community hospice, is quite different in some key areas. Institutional policies, financing, legal restrictions, unions, and differing departmental practices, all influence how volunteers are able to function and interact in this setting. This chapter looks at some of these variables and suggests ways to establish and enhance palliative care volunteer programmes in hospital settings. The authors have worked in different teaching hospitals of the same university and their experience at times has been similar and at times, very different, in accord with the culture and community bias of their respective hospitals. These similarities and differences will be highlighted to show the range of options for volunteer coordinators to design and implement volunteer palliative care programmes that address the specific needs and cultures of their institutions.

Guiding principles and assumptions

The role of the palliative care volunteer, in any setting, is to provide assistance, companionship, and support to terminally ill patients and their caregivers' or families. The aim of their involvement is to enhance the quality of life of the patient or caregiver by offering their time, practical support, commitment, and compassion throughout the illness experience. Our challenge is to offer such support within the complexities and boundaries of a large teaching hospital.

Two guiding principles and assumptions underscore the successful integration of volunteer programmes in hospital palliative care services and form the basis for ongoing communication with members of the professional palliative care team:

1 Volunteer programmes are an essential part of the hospital's palliative care service.

2 Volunteers are essential members of the interdisciplinary palliative care team.

These principles address the central question of whether volunteers are wanted, or needed, and in what capacity. If they are wanted, then by whom? The medical team? The nursing staff? What roles are they needed for? Are there union implications if volunteers are seen to be taking over staff roles, especially in times of budget constraints and downsizing of staff across the health-care spectrum? These are difficult and recurring questions for team management and their answers must be clearly established within the palliative care team and must be part of an ongoing dialogue as team members change. Flowing from these principles is a commitment from both the Volunteer Coordinator (or Volunteer Services Manager—VSM) and the members of the palliative care team to recognize and include the voice of volunteers in management meetings, decision making, patient rounds, and education programmes for all staff on the service. It is important for the VSM to develop clear standards of practice for volunteer services and to actively participate in quality assessment programmes and working groups within the hospital to ensure that the volunteer voice is heard and recognized as a key input to quality end-of-life care.

Administration: how the programme fits into the wider hospital framework

To whom is the programme accountable? To whom is each service component responsible? How are programme decisions made? What are the lines of reporting? Who controls and sets the budget? How does the programme fit into the wider volunteer framework within the hospital?

In a large teaching hospital, there are several volunteer departments, each with its own coordinator and volunteer team. In our hospitals, there are coordinators of volunteers in specialized departments, such as oncology, palliative care, emergency department, pastoral services, and there is an overall department of volunteers whose members perform a range of tasks including those in the gift shop, library, outpatient clinics, etc. It is essential that we coordinate programmes amongst ourselves to avoid overlap of service but retain continuity of service, for example, when a patient passes from an active treatment floor in oncology to the palliative care unit.

In our respective hospitals, we are accountable to the:

◆ Chief or administrative assistant of the palliative care service for day-to-day administration on the palliative care unit.

◆ Coordinator of the volunteer department of the hospital for issues that concern overall hospital policies and volunteer activities in the hospital.

We meet regularly with this person on hospital volunteer activities, report monthly on volunteer hours, process all applications through this office, keep them informed of any resignations, address changes, plan 'Volunteer Recognition Days' and activities with them, obtain parking passes, lunch tickets, and smocks and identification badges. This system works very well. It is important that we work with the volunteer department on general volunteer activities, but on issues that are pertinent to the palliative care unit, we need to work within the palliative care team and collaborate with other volunteer departments in the hospital as needed.

The interdisciplinary team/working together

It is the mantra of health-care systems that interdisciplinary teams provide the most comprehensive approach to patient care—each team member bringing a perspective and expertise that contributes to an understanding of the whole person.

What perspective and expertise does the volunteer bring to this team, and how will that voice be heard?

Whether you are establishing a new volunteer service or maintaining or expanding an existing one, it is essential to obtain an agreement from the palliative care team that volunteers are necessary, and that there is a clear mandate as to their role within the team:

- Establish guidelines for the volunteer programme—who will do what, when, and how? Will volunteers assist with patient care? Who will train them in this? To whom will volunteers report and how will they access patient information?

- A coordinator/manager (volunteer or paid) is needed to recruit, train, supervise, and liaise with volunteers, staff, and hospital administration.

- Examine, review, and become familiar with policies within the institution and its various departments on volunteers. Are there union constraints on what tasks volunteers can perform? Are there legal restrictions, for example, accessing or recording in patient charts? What insurance/liability coverage is available to volunteers who incur an injury on the job?

- New programmes must be negotiated through appropriate channels. Some are not always transferable; for example, pet therapy may work on one unit and not another for reasons of infection control.

- Volunteers must have ongoing training, support, and recognition. Recurrent debriefing, evaluation, and education is essential (by staff, coordinator, and other volunteers). Regular volunteer meetings provide a forum to discuss cases, share concerns, receive support from peers, and build a strong team.

- Volunteers must be given tools—information and feedback mechanisms such as tapes, record-keeping in notebooks, and direct communication with staff and coordinator. They must also be updated on any changes in infection protocols or other floor issues.

- Respect for volunteers from the team and from volunteers to the team is paramount. Volunteers should be accorded professional courtesies in line with their place on the multidisciplinary team and in turn, they need to follow through with commitment and responsibility to any task or patient to whom they are assigned.

- Develop a scheme to help volunteers cope with change. Teaching hospitals differ from smaller community hospitals in the frequency of staff changes. Volunteers must cope with frequent shift changes and changes of staff (residents, medical students on a short elective, fellows, research projects, etc.). Ongoing and reciprocal orientation to each other's work is necessary for effective communication.

Volunteers must follow rules, guidelines, and respect boundaries and confidences and these need to be clearly defined at interview and throughout training.

- Clear procedures for airing grievances and reporting incidents are essential.

- Individual talents and skills must be recognized and effectively utilized, keeping in mind that volunteers work under volunteer guidelines, not previous or external professional competencies.

◆ Clarity about financing and funding is essential. Who is financing the volunteer programme, including salary costs for the coordinator/manager, supplies, and materials? In both our hospitals, at present, the palliative care volunteer programme is privately resourced by donors, with office space and some supplies granted by the hospital administration. Fund-raising projects must be cleared with administration. It is imperative to establish clear goals and budget for the service and to work within this constraint.

◆ Information sharing. In both our services, patient information comes from the medical and nursing teams, patient charts, and attendance at ward rounds. Only accredited staff (including the volunteer coordinator) have access to patient records. (*Volunteers do not read nursing charts on patients and do not record in them.*) How is information about a patient passed to the volunteer? Our systems are different. In one hospital, information is verbally passed to the primary nurse and this is incorporated in a daily tape recording of information and instructions for volunteers, which is listened to by all volunteers as they start their shift. In another hospital, volunteers have their own log book, with separate entries for each patient. Staff have full access to these notes as do subsequent volunteers who can read brief notes about previous volunteer interactions and follow up on any individual requests. The volunteer notes do not form part of the hospital chart. Both systems work equally well, as does a general communication book where volunteers and staff can leave messages and notes to one another. The method of passing information is not prescribed; each coordinator and head nurse will determine a method which meets their needs for their unit and team.

◆ It is important that the volunteer coordinator meets regularly with unit staff and is involved in issues concerning the unit. A voice not heard is a voice easily overlooked.

Volunteer profile: who are the volunteers?

Volunteers are as mixed and varied as the patients and families they serve. They are the 82-year-old grandmother who has given a lifetime of service to others; the 38-year-old student completing a doctorate in languages; the 58-year-old retired social worker, herself a cancer survivor; the 66-year-old retired pharmacist; the 45-year-old mother returning to university to study psychology; the 56-year-old retired nurse, now a massage therapist; the immigrant mother wanting to help her community; the accountant wanting to work evenings, or the medical student wanting experience. Many faces, cultures, religions, and professions—they reflect the make-up of our multicultural and diverse community. Many have been touched by cancer—either personally or a close member of the family. Many have a personal affiliation and loyalty to the hospital where they choose to volunteer—they were born there; their father died there; they see it as their family hospital. Volunteers who are attracted to working in a hospital setting are often more educated and many have had experience in health-care settings, often in a professional capacity. Many students (particularly of medicine, nursing, and social work) apply to the programme looking for volunteer experience to supplement their résumé. They are often attracted by the prestige of the institution and staff and the educational opportunities to be found at a particular hospital. While their enthusiasm is infectious, they do not always remain with the programme and their class schedules can be a logistical nightmare for the volunteer coordinator.

The demographic profile of volunteers has changed in recent years. We do not have as many full-time homemakers who have made volunteering a part of their lives. Nowadays, these women are working and raising a family. We have many more working people who want to volunteer in the evenings and weekends (the coordinator usually works day shifts). Again, their schedules change frequently and they are often absent because of work or travel. More men are volunteering, but we need more. Many retirees now spend a significant part of the winter in warmer climates, thus also leaving gaps in scheduling and consistency of service. It is a constant challenge to recruit and retain a volunteer team that truly reflects the diversity of our patients and which will give reliable and consistent service without constantly amending the schedule.

We also attract many retired professionals. Among our volunteers we have retired physicians, social workers, physiotherapists, psychologists, nurses, a speech therapist, massage therapists, and business executives. From the outset it is necessary to fully explain that they must set their professional 'cap' aside. They are not there to mediate, diagnose, treat, or give advice, but to offer compassion and support. They are required to follow our rules and guidelines. Generally, they say they are relieved to not carry the responsibility of a professional, but happy just to accompany the patient and family—a luxury they did not have in a professional capacity.

In our hospitals, it would not be possible for an active health-care professional to work, in their professional capacity, as a volunteer, with the exception of some complementary therapists, such as a massage therapist or aromatherapist. These therapists often donate a few hours per week, and in both our hospitals receive referrals receive referrals from the medical and nursing teams, via the head nurse or the VSM. They are part of the Voluntary Service and subject to the same screening, as well as their professional qualifications being accepted by the Chief of the Division. While health professionals do not work as volunteers, it must be said that everyone on the team—doctors, nurses, psychologists, etc., regularly work hours over and above their paid duties, come to the hospital after-hours or on days off to sit with a patient, attend a celebration which is meaningful to a family, or to make condolence visits. While they are not volunteers in any literal sense, they share much in spirit. It is what makes a good team work—knowing that team members will do what is necessary in the interests of patients and their colleagues.

Recruitment and selection of volunteers

Selection must be thorough and careful as in all palliative care settings. Special considerations in a teaching hospital setting are:

- ◆ Recruitment should target a good representative mix of ages, cultures, experience, and languages if possible to meet the needs of patients in a multicultural hospital.
- ◆ Volunteers in a hospital setting must be team players and respect boundaries, guidelines of the programme, institution, and departments.

◆ Volunteers need to be screened and accepted both by the palliative care VSM and the coordinator of volunteers for the hospital. The initial interview provides the opportunity for the coordinator to explore and assess the applicant's motives, expectations, suitability, and stability. There are many motivations for volunteering in a palliative unit, including the wish to 'give back' if their loved one had the experience of receiving good palliative care or wanting to give to others what had not been available to them when they needed it. Some feel it is part of their own personal growth journey. Our aim, as volunteer coordinators, is to ensure that an applicant's personal agenda, including their religious beliefs or a need to ease past losses, does not interfere with, or compromise, a patient's well-being and personal values. In our hospitals, a police check is also required.

◆ Volunteers must wear appropriate identification at all times—smock or coat and name badge.

A day in the life of a volunteer in Montreal: what do they do?

Assuming the volunteer has passed the initial interview and completed the compulsory training programme, what is expected of them on any given day?

◆ First and foremost, they listen. They are there for the patient and family to support them in any way possible. A conversation, accompaniment in silence, a gentle hand or foot massage, tidying the room, offering a cup of tea—all are small ways to ease the burden of the patient or family member and provide a moment of 'normality' in an otherwise noisy and busy hospital environment.

◆ Assist the nurse with patient care. Volunteers are assigned in the morning to work with the nurses helping to change beds, give bed baths, showers, and whirlpool baths, help with feeding (from delivery of trays to total feeding), personal care, toileting, transferring, massage, etc. Volunteers are kept informed about 'do's and don'ts' by means of a comprehensive daily report from the nurse. Transfers are never done alone, and all care is done under the supervision of the nurse. Training is provided in areas of transfers, feeding, infection control, and mobilization. Volunteers never give medication or do any medical interventions (injections, dressing changes, catheter insertions, etc.). However, they are often present to assist in some way (holding hands, supporting the patient, fetching supplies, handing the nurse equipment, etc.).

◆ Take patients for a walk or in a wheelchair, or help with recreation and hobbies, where appropriate.

◆ Provide respite to a tired caregiver. Volunteers may sit with a patient while a caregiver goes for lunch or runs personal errands.

◆ Provide a link to the team. Volunteers often hear and see things that may be relevant to the patient's care plan, particularly how much pain is being experienced or expressed to staff—'they're so busy!'. A volunteer may encourage the patient to report symptoms or pain to the doctor, or with their permission, pass on relevant information to staff. Volunteers have an important advocacy role both for patients and families.

Volunteers bring care, compassion, and companionship to those to whom they are assigned. They bring themselves—their personalities, quirks, stories, experience, wit, and wisdom and mostly they bring the gift of time. In a busy tertiary referral teaching hospital where staff rush from patient to patient and complaints about 'not having enough time' to spend with patients are common, volunteers take the time to make a difference in someone's day. It is not uncommon for volunteers to do special things for a patient, bring in a video of a hockey game to watch with a patient, help someone make a scrapbook, teach someone to knit, or to bring special treats and homemade goodies. Sometimes a patient needs to be careful what he/she wishes for—a loose remark of 'I just want some chicken soup' soon has the unit awash in chicken soup as each volunteer brings enough to start a small restaurant. Staff can eat very well sometimes from the generosity of volunteers!

Volunteers help with the many personal events and celebrations on the palliative care unit. We have assisted and witnessed many birthdays, holiday celebrations, baptisms, bar mitzvahs, and weddings—each helping a patient or family member achieve a meaningful goal in their life. Volunteers provide music, food, and any special assistance to make the event personal and memorable. Most events are small in size, but recently we had a full wedding reception, highlighting the need for co-operation between multiple departments of the hospital to make it happen. One of our patients wanted to see the last of his children married and it was obvious that he would not live to the pre-planned date. The family decided to bring the wedding forward and have the ceremony and a small reception on the unit. Some sixty guests were planned and this could not be accommodated on the unit. So, quick planning between the volunteers, the hospital chaplain, house-keeping, recreation, and the nursing staff on the geriatrics unit resulted in a wedding being held on this unit, where there was more space, and a full wedding, complete with bridesmaids, photographer, caterers, and a three-piece band was possible. We were able to help a very proud father witness and give blessings to the marriage of his daughter, enjoy a dance in his bed with his wife and daughter and to capture the moment for future generations. It was a day of grace and love, and it brought together staff and volunteers from different services who were also blessed by the moment.

Volunteers do not plan weddings on an everyday basis!—but they are part of many small meaningful moments for patients and their families. It is what they do best and for what they are most appreciated, and it is always a surprise what might happen on any given day.

Where do the volunteers work?

Volunteers work all over the hospital, in every department and clinic. The volunteers in the wider hospital fall under the supervision of the Coordinator of Volunteers for the hospital who has a separate staff. There are many volunteer activities from a 'cuddles programme' in the neonatal department to volunteers in the transplant and dialysis departments. All require separate applications and training programmes and generally there is no integration of volunteers.

Palliative care volunteers must apply, be accepted, and be trained to be part of the palliative care team. They work in the following areas.

Palliative care unit

Volunteers work primarily on the unit itself—a 16–17 bed-dedicated unit. Shifts are normally 4 hours each, although some volunteers choose to work longer hours. Morning, afternoon, and evening shifts are offered, 7 days a week.

Oncology floors

Palliative care volunteers are not loaned to other departments when there is a shortfall or high need, but palliative care volunteers do visit patients on other floors, at the referral of the consulting team. These patients are often on a waiting list for admission to the palliative unit, and it significantly reduces the stress of patients and families to know a familiar face and have a relationship with a volunteer if the patient is ultimately admitted to the unit. Many families tell us it made all the difference and allayed a great deal of fear about the unit itself. Sometimes, the referral is for a patient who will remain on another floor, at the recommendation of their physician, even if a bed on the unit becomes available. In this case, the volunteer would 'visit' and provide support, perhaps assist with feeding, but would not be part of the team on that floor, per se. The volunteer is part of the palliative care team, in this case providing outreach to a patient on another floor.

Bereavement outreach

Some volunteers also work in bereavement outreach and support programmes. Volunteers who have themselves experienced a loss and have completed special training, may be matched with a newly bereaved person and call them at regular intervals over a period of 12 months, until the first anniversary of the death.

Other volunteers, also specially trained, co-lead bereavement support groups, which are offered in 8-week sessions several times a year. The bereavement volunteers receive referrals, support, and direction from a bereavement coordinator, who may be the same person as the Palliative Care Coordinator (VSM), or not. Both models exist in our hospitals. The important factor is that bereavement is seen as an essential part of the palliative care programme and volunteers are a key element of the service.

Ecumenical memorial services

In conjunction with pastoral services, a memorial service is offered on the palliative care unit, at intervals appropriate for the institution, for families who have lost a loved one. Volunteers and staff are invited to this service and volunteers play an active role in hosting a tea at the end of the service. Members of the bereavement team are present to assist families, especially those who are alone or seem isolated in their grief.

Training and ongoing education

Training is the cornerstone of the volunteer programme and provides it with credibility and professionalism. It is compulsory for all volunteers to complete a comprehensive training programme before they start work on the service. (See Appendix 1.) It changes a little from year to year to reflect new topics and concerns. For example, 'Ethics' and 'Complementary Therapies' are relatively recent additions. In addition, there is an expectation that volunteers will avail themselves of regular in-house education opportunities to enhance their skills. Further areas of training include:

◆ Practical training in admission criteria for palliative care, diseases involved, treatment options, DNR (Do Not Resuscitate) orders, hydration, feeding, palliative surgery, radiotherapy and chemotherapy, infection control procedures, transfers, feeding, personal hygiene care, and mobilization techniques.

◆ Volunteers must be thoroughly oriented to working on the unit and in other departments in the hospital. This can be done by an experienced volunteer.

◆ A clearly defined probation period, mentoring with an experienced volunteer, and scheduled time with the VSM for debriefing and feedback are important training practices.

◆ In our services, the formal training programme is usually provided by professionals on the palliative care service. During the year, staff may also be invited to lecture to the volunteers on a given topic, and volunteers are always invited to university palliative care rounds or to hear visiting lecturers. Volunteers are very much included in educational activities and conferences, which provide networking opportunities with other volunteers from different settings.

◆ Volunteer team meetings once a month are another rich source of training and support.

Training for staff

Training must also be provided for staff to sensitize them to working with volunteers. This is an extremely important area and one that is often overlooked. In a teaching hospital, this needs to be done on a frequent basis to accommodate changing rotations of residents and medical students.

Common problems and special issues

Having briefly highlighted some of the factors necessary to establish and maintain a professionally accepted and professional volunteer programme in a large teaching hospital, we now look at some of the most common problems we have encountered in coordinating our teams:

◆ *Selecting and retaining appropriate volunteers*—often the most keen, enthusiastic applicants are those who do not last—the job does not meet the expectations they had of it, or their personal schedule is too demanding to allow consistency of volunteering. During the interview and the training one can weed out some inappropriate volunteers, and the probation period provides a good opportunity for close supervision.

◆ *Finding appropriate tasks for volunteers who have special skills and experience*, including using them as mentors or buddies to other volunteers. Developing a skills' bank is one way to keep track of the special talents of individual volunteers.

◆ *Juggling schedules and being flexible enough to accommodate volunteers' schedules*—some volunteers are away for the whole summer, or the whole winter, students' schedules change frequently, volunteers take vacations or are sick.

◆ *Finding creative ways to train volunteers* and to keep the in-house education updated and appropriate to the knowledge and skill level of the volunteers, especially for veteran volunteers with many years of experience.

◆ *Providing ongoing feedback and support to volunteers to enhance their skills.* This can be a full-time job in itself, but one which pays huge dividends in retaining volunteers and preventing major disciplinary problems.

◆ *Recognizing and dealing with grief and potential 'burnout' of team members*—providing support, a leave of absence, if appropriate, and follow-up.

◆ *Increasing the demand for volunteer services only to find there are not sufficient volunteers* or conversely, having too many volunteers and not enough work. This is a rare occurrence but speaks to the need for ongoing communication with the palliative care team to ensure that staff, particularly new staff, are aware of the volunteer's role and relevant availability and can therefore make appropriate requests for volunteers to assist with a patient or family member.

◆ *Expanding and developing the volunteer programme when professional staff are being 'downsized' by the institution as a result of budget constraints.* This is a new challenge for VSMs and it will only increase as health systems undergo reform and change. The possibility of 'turf wars' is an area of great sensitivity and requires honest communication, trust, and clear definition of roles and responsibilities within the whole palliative care team. It may be necessary to meet with union representation if a threat to their jobs is perceived.

In many ways, it is an anomaly to have a palliative care unit in an acute care hospital, where the ethos is cure, rapid processing of patients, and releasing beds as soon as possible. Volunteers working on the palliative unit are somewhat protected from this pressure, but it is certainly felt on oncology floors where patients are treated, discharged, and re-admitted as needed. It is more difficult to build relationships with the patients and families and the volunteer may pass by the room many times before connecting with a patient who is having tests or treatment. Even on the palliative care unit, there may be multiple admissions as a patient's pain and symptoms are managed (sometimes with radiation, chemotherapy, or surgery for palliative relief of the symptoms); the patient may go home for a while and be re-admitted if the symptoms again cause a level of distress that cannot be managed with home care.

In our hospitals today, there is often a shortage of nurses and beds, and there are long waiting lists, including for palliative care. Volunteers can and do find this stressful at times, but it is the role of the VSM to debrief with volunteers they assess as being noticeably stressed or at risk of burnout, and 'Taking Care of Oneself' is a training module repeated as often as required.

Dismissing a volunteer

Dealing with volunteers who overstep guidelines and boundaries can be challenging. Is it ever necessary to dismiss a volunteer? Have we ever had to do so? If a volunteer were to overstep a boundary (e.g. giving aromatherapy to a patient without approval), we would sit with that volunteer to explain the implications of doing this and to re-emphasize the importance of following the rules and checking with the staff before doing so. There may be allergies, respiratory problems, etc., of which the volunteer is unaware. Generally, this would be sufficient, and can be set in a context of ongoing training and support for the volunteer. However, if it happened again it would be much more serious and the volunteer would probably be asked to leave.

It is seldom necessary to dismiss volunteers but volunteers may be counselled to leave if they are becoming over-involved with patients and not having a clear sense of personal boundaries. This may indicate unresolved issues or loss in their own past and the emotional nature of palliative care work may not suit them. A different volunteer experience, in a less stressful part of the hospital or community may be more suited to their needs. Sometimes, we recommend a volunteer take a leave of absence from the programme to prevent burnout and take some time for themselves.

We would ask a volunteer to leave if they have been consistently unreliable in reporting for work. Usually, this indicates a lack of enthusiasm or availability for the job and, as we generally have a waiting list for volunteer positions, we will give the spot to another. In many years it has not happened very often. We start with the assumption that the volunteer is well-intentioned and we find that good screening, training, mentoring by an experienced volunteer, and ongoing communication and support for the volunteer during the probation period works well and prevents most problems becoming major ones.

Challenges and opportunities for the VSM

Healthcare is changing; downsizing is a reality, and the volunteer role is more important than ever. VSMs are faced with great challenges and opportunities to introduce innovative programmes to supplement those of the medical and nursing teams. But it can be a lonely job, often poorly financed, if at all, and with many more tasks to fill the day than hours allowed. We offer a few suggestions that have helped us in our work and have offered us inspiration, joy, and challenge.

Network with others

This is possibly the single most effective way to broaden your perspective and experience. Link with other volunteer coordinators in your community—hospitals, hospices, and community health programmes. Meet on a regular basis (e.g. every other month), and share programme ideas, upcoming workshops and seminars, challenges and concerns, and even more importantly, your successes. The support of your peers is enriching and invaluable and in a very practical sense, can save you time and money by sharing resources, advertising each other's workshops, and developing some common training materials. The network does not need to be exclusively palliative care. In Montreal, we have developed a rich network of volunteer coordinators/ VSMs from oncology day programmes as well as those in palliative care. Where the opportunity does not exist for personal contact with other coordinators, this can be done online, for example. The important thing is to link with others and share ideas and experience.

Share the training

As mentioned earlier, there is much to be gained by sharing resources, expenses, and ideas with other coordinators. In recent years, we have joined with the coordinator of another hospital in Montreal and the three of us have devised a common training programme, based on the standards of the Canadian Palliative Care Association. Similar standards are available in many countries. We have presented this material in three different formats to meet the needs of our hospitals and the volunteer applicants:

◆ A 2-day weekend workshop
◆ A 4-evening workshop (2 evenings per week)
◆ A 2-day mid-week workshop

Each hospital provided trainers and volunteers, and material costs were shared. Each of these formats was highly interactive and experiential in design. Role-plays, discussions, and hands-on practice of hygiene care, for example, were key features. These inter-hospital programmes supplemented existing lecture-based training in each hospital. Feedback from participants showed that the inter-hospital format was highly successful in encouraging networking, and exploring differences between hospitals, particularly cultural and religious differences between some individual programmes and the differences in roles performed by the volunteers in different settings. Some were more hands-on, assisting with bed care and personal hygiene, with other hospitals adopting a more 'friendly visitor' role for their volunteers.

Sharing training also meant that more volunteers could be trained on a regular basis, rather than each hospital waiting until they had 'enough' to justify the expense of running their own training programme. A further benefit was that it met volunteers' personal needs more quickly—they were able to start work sooner, and could get a training programme to suit their hours. Full-time workers appreciated the evening or weekend schedules, and others, particularly retired people, appreciated the day-time hours.

Be informed

Read current journals and articles. There is a growing wealth of literature in volunteer management in general, both in print and on the Internet. Explore relevant Web sites for free ideas on training, management, programme design, and volunteer recognition ideas, to name but a few. Contribute to on-line discussions about your work and learn from others in similar settings.

Use the resources of the team

Although the interdisciplinary team model is so prized, its full resources are often not used, and problem-solving in isolation is common. Fellow team members may have a perspective, experience, and insight that are valuable and relevant to the issue you are dealing with, whether it be training, discipline, administration, scheduling, or emotional support for yourself or one of your volunteer team. Use your team members—it builds trust, camaraderie, and interdependence—as well as possibly solving your problem. Equally, valuable resources exist within your volunteer team. Use them. It is an excellent way to identify potential leaders, mentors, and trainers.

Participate in hospital committees and rounds

Teaching hospitals abound in committees and working groups. The volunteer voice is best heard when it is part of multidisciplinary committees—for example, committees and working groups on Palliative Care Standards, Bereavement, Quality of Life, Pastoral Care, and Humanization of Care, and is most easily overlooked when it is not represented. The VSM should be involved, participating actively in ward rounds and ad hoc meetings of ward personnel.

Take advantage of teaching opportunities

One thing teaching hospitals obviously do is teach, and there are many opportunities for VSMs to contribute. They can offer to present the volunteer perspective and role at orientations for new nurses and residents. This is a valuable and ongoing opportunity for dialogue with other disciplines, as staff regularly change rotations in a teaching facility. Present a case at rounds or take advantage of Theme weeks such as Volunteer Week, Palliative Care Week, Humanization of Care Week, etc., to present the volunteer perspective. The organizing committees of such events are always looking for lectures, seminars, and workshops of interest, and it is both a challenge and an opportunity for volunteers to have their voice heard.

In the same vein, participate in local, national, and international conferences where possible, and advocate for a volunteer forum as part of the conference agenda. Networking, teaching, and learning with others is a rich way to broaden one's knowledge and contribute to a developing field of practice wisdom. Encourage volunteers to attend, if the budget allows, and have them present their learning to the next team meeting or write a summary for the team newsletter.

Plan for the future

An annual review of goals and objectives, both for the programme as well as for individual volunteers allows the VSM to keep focus on what is needed to develop his/her programme as well as to devise a strategy to raise funds or solicit donors, as necessary. Have a 'Vision Day'—put on some 3-D glasses and discover if you are seeing clearly!

Are you meeting the needs of the unit, the volunteers (how do you know—have you asked them lately?) Evaluations and surveys (formal or informal) are extremely important and informative. Are you meeting your own needs? What needs to change, if anything?

Follow the 3-D approach:

◆ Delete when necessary.

◆ Delegate whenever possible.

◆ Dream about the day when volunteer departments are adequately funded and resourced and you can take it easy!

Conclusion

Despite its sometimes difficult moments, the authors of this chapter have rarely been disenchanted with their work. It has been a joy and a privilege to work in this field and it will become only richer and more exciting as VSMs share their skills and experience and help develop global standards for our work. It is a challenge and a great opportunity for us all.

Appendix 1

A typical training programme (names of speakers deleted)

Volunteer Training Programme—2001

This training programme is open to all new and current Palliative Care Service and McGill affiliated hospital staff and Volunteers and interested members of the public.

SESSION I:
6:30–7:30
7:45–9:00

THURSDAY, SEPTEMBER 20, 2001
The Role of the Volunteer
The Philosophy of Palliative Care

SESSION II:
6:30–7:30
7:45–9:00

THURSDAY, SEPTEMBER 27, 2001
Nursing in Palliative Care
Pain Management

SESSION III:
6:30–7:30
7:45–9:00

THURSDAY, OCTOBER 4, 2001
Families Facing Death
Music Therapy in Palliative Care

SESSION IV:
6:30–7:30
7:45–9:00

THURSDAY, OCTOBER 11, 2001
Quality of Life for Palliative Care Patients and Their Families
Pastoral Care for Palliative Patients and Their Families

SESSION V:
6:30–7:30
7:45–9:00

THURSDAY, OCTOBER 18, 2001
Bereavement Follow-Up in Palliative care
The Volunteer Experience

SESSION VI:
6:30–7:30
7:45–9:00

THURSDAY, OCTOBER 25, 2001
Occupational Therapy in Palliative Care
Complimentary and Alternative Therapies in Palliative Care

SESSION VII:
6:30–7:30
7:45–9:00

THURSDAY, NOVEMBER 1, 2001
Ethics in Palliative Care
Psychology in Palliative Care

Chapter 16

Neighbourhood Network in Palliative Care, Kerala, India

Dr Suresh Kumar

Palliative care programmes in the south Indian state of Kerala have attracted a good amount of international attention on different counts. These include: the estimated good coverage for palliative care and long-term care in a 'resource poor' setting, the enthusiasm that has been generated in the local community, the reliance on locally generated funds, and the good potential for sustainability[1–5]. In this programme called Neighbourhood Network in Palliative Care (NNPC), volunteers from the local community are trained to identify problems of the chronically ill in their area and to intervene effectively, with active support from a network of trained professionals. Management and coordination of the programme is also by community volunteers.

Kerala—the background

Before moving on to discuss the programme in more detail, it may be helpful to understand the wider context in which NNPC exists. Kerala is the southernmost state in India with an area of 39,000 sq. km and a population of 32 million. It consists of only 1.18 per cent of the country's land area and 3.4 per cent of the population. Kerala had attracted good international attention and many researchers in the past owing to its remarkable achievements in health, despite poor economic growth. Kerala has exceptionally good health indicators, such as crude death rate, infant mortality rate, and life expectancy, putting the region on a par with many developed nations. The high statistical achievements in health on the background of low per capita income were first brought to international attention through a publication in 1975 by a group of economists[6]. Kerala achieved the health status as par with that of USA spending roughly $10 per capita per year while United States spends about $3500 per capita per year on health care. Kerala's high health status in terms of standard health indicators, with comparatively low governmental spending in health-care services, has prompted many analysts to suggest that this 'Kerala Model' is worth emulating by other developing regions of the world.

Different explanations have been given for this phenomenon. Leading interpretations emphasize factors such as the unique socio-political environment in the state, high basic health awareness due to high literacy level, an extensive and efficient public health-care system, and higher accessibility to healthcare due to better infrastructure at the local level[7]. The state has also created equality of access to healthcare regardless of class, caste, gender, and regional considerations[8]. Public provisions of education and health and equitable access to these services have been the twin founding pillars of the Kerala model. Substantial social security entitlements to help vulnerable sections of society have served to further strengthen the egalitarian base of Kerala's development.

A comparison of the share of medical and public health services shows that, in Kerala, health services (including medical and public health services) always had a consistently higher percentage share than the rest of India until the end of 1980s. Since then, the difference between Kerala and the other states in the percentage share of health services has declined. The public expenditure on health and family welfare which reached 11.67 per cent as a percentage of State Domestic Product (SDP) by 1983–1984 fell to 9.94 per cent in 1989–1990 and declined further to 6.36 per cent in 2005–2006. The social security entitlements which, as a percentage of SDP, were increasing at a rate of 1.83 per cent during the pre-reform period, also fell to 0.15 per cent during the reform regime. Poor-quality education and healthcare have been the net outcome of this. The process of exclusion of low-income groups from access to good-quality healthcare due to its increasing commercialization was compounded by cuts to public spending. A recent study has shown that around 14 per cent of individuals in rural, and 11 per cent in urban, Kerala incurred expenditure on health-care in excess of 15 per cent of their income and that these 'catastrophic expenses' were concentrated mostly among the poor. It has pushed 3.8 per cent individuals in rural, and 4.5 per cent in urban, Kerala below the poverty line[9].

The expansion of the private sector, particularly in rural areas, to fill the vacuum created by the retreating government has a definite bearing on the cost of healthcare. The rapidly increasing health-care expenditure in Kerala is detrimentally affecting the access of the poor to healthcare, as the escalating costs of private services and reduced public investments generate inequalities. A recent study on outpatient care utilization in urban Kerala points to these inequalities in access despite the expansion of private healthcare[10]. People with chronic, incurable, and terminal illness are usually the most seriously affected among the population having no or limited access to healthcare.

Palliative care in Kerala—the beginning

Kerala had pain clinics in two cancer centres in 1990. But the first palliative care initiative in region was started in 1993[11]. The unit had an outpatient clinic and home care services in a structure very similar to most palliative care/hospice programmes in the west. The community's participation was limited to involvement of a few volunteers in nursing and associated roles within the institution and to donation of money[12,13]. The service was provided by a few doctors and offered symptom relief and emotional support to those who attended the outpatient clinic. The home care service acted as a patchy extension of the clinical support to limited regions in the community[14]. In the first few years, the organization also tried to establish this model of care in the surrounding areas. Satellite centres were set up in the nearby areas. Although some of the resources came from the community, involvement of the local community in policy/management was minimal. These early palliative care clinics were essentially services initiated by a few health-care professionals to care for incurable patients in the area. The recognition of the inadequacies of this model both in terms of coverage and other dimensions of total care led to a lot of discussions and experiments at the organizational level.

Neighbourhood Network in Palliative Care (NNPC)

Attempts to develop a community-owned service, addressing the defects of the earlier model were strengthened by the formal initiation of a project, the Neighbourhood Network in Palliative Care (NNPC), in the district of Malappuram in 2001, by four organizations—two already working in palliative care and two working in other areas of social work.

The programme, aimed at the development of a sustainable cost-effective system of care for the incurable and terminally ill patients with community participation, had its focus at grass roots level. The strategy was to encourage local people to address the social needs of the patients and families, train the community volunteers to offer emotional support, facilitate the development of locally sustainable home care programmes, and to establish a network of nurses and doctors with expertise in palliative care to support these initiatives. The programme was enthusiastically received by the community. Within 7 years, the initiative grew into a vast network of 74 community-owned palliative care programmes looking after more than 8000 patients at any point of time. It has a workforce of more than 5000 trained community volunteers, more than 50 palliative care physicians and more than 100 palliative care nurses. Patients and their families are not charged for any service offered. This community-owned network of palliative care initiatives is now probably the largest palliative care network in the world.

NNPC does not aim to replace health-care professionals with volunteers. Instead, what is being attempted is to supplement the efforts of trained doctors and nurses in psychosocial and spiritual support by trained volunteers in the community. Groups of trained volunteers are tied to Palliative Care professionals and health-care facilities in their communities. The action plans clearly define the roles and responsibilities of individuals and institutions[15].

Community volunteers in NNPC

Any person willing to spend more than 2 hours every week to care for the chronically or incurably ill people in their village, can become a community volunteer in NNPC. Those who register are given a 15 hour structured training at the 'entry point'. Topics covered include the basics of palliative care, communication skills, emotional support, basic nursing skills, and organizational aspects of care. Prospective volunteers also make home visits as part of the training with the home care team led by a nurse or doctor. Those who successfully complete the training are enrolled as community volunteers in NNPC. Trained volunteers form local groups to develop palliative care services in their locality.

Volunteers registered belong to all walks of life. Manual labourers, housewives, students, teachers, small-time farmers, merchants, and pensioners form the major part of the group. A good percentage of the volunteers have experience of social or political work. The majority are people who belong to poor or lower-middle socio-economic class.

Community volunteers in NNPC have been responsible for setting up most of the existing palliative care units in the network. The trained volunteers:

◆ Initiate and run palliative care units in their locality.

◆ Visit patients at home (both with the home care unit and on their own).

◆ Help at the outpatient clinic (Keeping the patients comfortable, talking to them, helping with clerking etc).

◆ Perform administrative work (including clerical work and account keeping).

◆ Raise funds for the unit; and

◆ Mobilize support for the patients from the various governmental and non-governmental agencies.

All the palliative care units in the network have palliative care physician-led outpatient clinic services in the region. The doctor–nurse team, which manages these outpatient clinics are employed by the local community volunteer groups. The number of out-patient clinic days per week varies from unit to unit. Patients registered at one unit can attend outpatient clinic run by other units also. Services offered by these clinics include:

◆ Medical consultations

◆ Medicines

◆ Procedures like tapping of ascetic fluids

◆ Wound care

Most patients are visited at home by community volunteers. In addition, all the units offer regular nurse-led home care services, supplemented by home visits by doctors. Services offered by the professional home care units include:

◆ Medical/nursing consultations.

◆ Procedures like urinary bladder catheterization and sometimes tapping of ascetic fluids.

◆ Wound care.

In addition to the medical and nursing services offered, all the units in the network also offer:

◆ A regular supply of food for the starving families. This usually comes as a weekly supply of rice and other items collected from individuals and shops in the neigh-bourhood. 'Rice for the family' has become an important component of *total care* for patients in the region, as a good percentage of families are financially broken by the cost of prolonged treatment by the time the patient registers with the palliative care unit.

◆ Support for children from families of poor patients to continue their education. The support is mainly in the form of books, uniforms, and umbrella at the time of opening of the school. Since almost all these children study at schools run or aided by the government, where education is free, tuition fee is not an issue. Students, however, tend to drop out at the beginning of academic year because the parents are not able to afford the expenses on books and uniforms. Intervention by the palliative care units at that point keeps them going. A few students are also supported for their university education.

◆ Transport to referral hospitals. In most situations, this is in the form of a vehicle offered free of charge for a follow up visit/admission at the Medical College hospital in Calicut or for an admission at the Institute of Palliative Medicine at Calicut. The trip otherwise would cost the family a month's income.

◆ Rehabilitation. There is a regular attempt to encourage/train/support patients/ family members in income-generating activities. The programmes include support/ training in making handicrafts, paper bags/envelopes etc., and support in rearing chicken, keeping cattle, and setting up small shops. Training workshops are organized for patients and family members.

◆ Financial support. Most units offer occasional financial support to the very poor patients in emergency situations.

◆ Emotional Support. Community volunteers trained in psychosocial support interact with patients and family to offer emotional support.

All the units also try to link their patients with local social or religious organizations supporting the marginalized.

Palliative Care units in the network also act as the link between the patient and the local government to help the patient to get benefits from government schemes. These include support for the destitute, electricity connection to homes of cancer patients, pension for cancer patients, etc.

Institute of Palliative Medicine

The Institute of Palliative Medicine is the nodal centre for NNPC. The institute, in collaboration with the district level committees addresses the quality control and training requirements of the network. It also acts as the policy, research, and training arm of the WHO Demonstration project in palliative care for the Developing World.

The Institute of Palliative Medicine also runs regular training courses in palliative care for health-care professionals. Trainees include doctors and nurses from all over South East Asia.

The 30-bed inpatient unit at the Institute offers admission to patients registered with any unit in the network. Admission can be for symptom relief, terminal care, or respite for the family. Any doctor, nurse, or community volunteer in the network can refer patients, but a discussion by telephone with the nurse or doctor on duty is necessary to confirm the objective of admission, provisional management plan, and availability of beds.

Fund-raising

Funds for the activities of the units are generated through donations from individuals and institutions. Donation boxes kept at public places are a major source of income. Seventy-five per cent of the individual donations are of amounts less than 30 pence. All the units also receive support from the local government, which is estimated to be one-third of the total expenditure in the case of most units in the network. Other sources of income include small regular donations from school children, donations from non-residential Indians (employed in Gulf countries), and donations from crew of the buses from the nearby bus stations.

The Institute of Palliative Medicine has also received grants from various international agencies.

New initiatives under the NNPC umbrella

An interesting recent occurrence has been the development of various closely related initiatives under the NNPC umbrella. These include projects to support needy patient populations who are generally not covered by conventional palliative care and are described briefly in the following paragraphs.

Pariraksha

Pariraksha is a joint venture by the District Panchayat (local government) in Malappuram and NNPC groups in the district to establish panchayat level home care programmes with community participation to support and guide all the chronically and incurably ill patients in the district. The 3-year programme, once established, will be supporting and keeping track of more than 20 000 patients. Institute of Palliative Medicine provides technical support for the project.

Malappuram Initiative in Community Psychiatry

Malappuram Initiative in Community Psychiatry is a much-appreciated project to take care of the chronic psychiatric patients in the community. The project is run by a group of community volunteers from palliative care in collaboration with the Calicut-based Institute of Mental Health and Neurosciences.

Kidney Patient Welfare Society

Kidney Patient Welfare Societies in Malappuram and Kozhikode Districts in Kerala are charities formed by NNPC volunteers to support post-transplant patients and patients on chronic dialysis.

Care 4 Childhood Cancer and Chronic Illness (C4CCCI)

The number of children accessing palliative care in Kerala is only a fraction of those in need of it. A group of palliative care volunteers in Calicut formed a charity to support children with chronic illness through their both curative and palliative phase of treatment. The organization acts also as the link between Institute of Palliative Medicine and the Department of Paediatrics at Calicut Medical College.

Organizational activities

A fairly good percentage of volunteers have been social or political activists in the past. Many continue these activities along with the community volunteer work in palliative care. This has resulted in the availability of exceptionally good organizational skills in the palliative care network. Organizing awareness and training programmes in the community and advocacy work with the local governments and other agencies are important components of the activities of NNPC. Most of the sessions in training programmes for new volunteers are also led by experienced volunteers from the network. Community volunteers in NNPC have established a definite identity of their own in Kerala's social sphere. Annual state level conferences of community volunteers in palliative care have been held every year for the last 5 years.

The Government of Kerala has declared its palliative care policy in 2008, achieving the distinction of being the first government in the region to do so. The policy endorses the role of community volunteers in palliative care, accepts the government's responsibility in providing palliative care, and sets an action plan for the development of palliative care services by local governments with community participation[22].

Discussion

Neighbourhood Network in Palliative Care is therefore characterized by

- A massive well-knit network of community volunteers at grass roots level.
- A collective rather than individual approach to palliative care.
- A social rather than medical model of health and diseases.
- Participation of community members in health-care decisions. Massive involvement of the community volunteers is seen at all levels of care including need assessment, planning. and delivery.
- Need-based as against diagnosis-based services. The network offers medical, nursing and psychosocial help to all patients with incurable illness irrespective of the diagnosis.
- Emphasis on home-based care.

What makes the initiative different from palliative care projects in many other regions of the world is the extent and depth of community intervention. The programme is very much in line with the WHO Declaration of Alma Ata—'Health for All' through primary healthcare: 'Primary healthcare is essential healthcare based on appropriate and acceptable methods and technology made universally available to individuals and families in the community through their full participation and at a cost that the community and country can afford to maintain in the spirit of self-reliance'[16]. It has been mentioned that this community approach in palliative care, 28 years after Alma Ata, shows the way forward for palliative care to 'Palliative Care for All'[4].

Community participation in different programmes is usually of two types depending on the perspectives[17]. What most programmes (including the majority of Palliative Care programmes) mean by community participation is only utilization of community resources (money, manpower, etc.) to supplement what is otherwise available for the programme. Volunteers in such programmes are asked to fill certain preset 'slots'. They do not play any major role in planning, evaluating, monitoring, or modifying the programme. On the other hand, community participation can also be a tool for empowerment, enabling local communities to take responsibility for identifying and working together to solve their own health and developmental problems. NNPC can be seen as an attempt at such a community development programme in Palliative Care.

The community is diverse, with wide differences in socioeconomic status, educational status, religion, ethnicity, and so on. Because different groups in a community have widely differing needs and priorities, participatory projects can have different impacts in a range of areas[18]. The extent of participation of people from the poor and lower-middle-class strata of the society has been one of the main characteristics of the NNPC programme[19]. NNPC is also working closely with the local governments in many places, engaging them to identify and prioritize the local health needs[20]. For example, in the district of Malappuram, locally called the 'laboratory for NNPC', more than 30 per cent of funds for the palliative care activities came as a contribution from the local government. 'Pariraksha', a comprehensive home care programme for the bedridden, initiated by the local government in Malappuram, has been developed in collaboration with NNPC in that district. Funding for this innovative programme comes from the local governments in the district as well as government of Kerala's 'Arogyakeralam' (Healthy Kerala) project.

Kerala has a history of very successful social movements. The social movements in the nineteenth century and early twentieth century were aimed against caste-based discrimination. Since the 1930s, Kerala also witnessed a strong trade union and socialist movements[21]. A history of a widespread library movement, a strong popular science movement, and a recent literacy movement makes Kerala different from other states in India. What Kerala had, essentially, was a strong political society that mediated between the people and the state, which successfully presented the demands for the basic amenities of life to the state. The massive grass roots level participation and collective action rather than individual voluntary initiatives makes NNPC also more of a social movement than a simple community volunteer programme. This, beyond volunteerism, is about confidence-building for the individual within the group and from the group to the individual. People from the lower-middle and poor social class form the bulk of the NNPC volunteers. This is the same social group to which majority of the patients cared for by the programme also belong. This active involvement of people in issues that affect their lives gives this palliative care programme a unique community development dimension. The rapid development of the initiative is happening at a time when Kerala's equity-based health and education systems have started showing signs of failure under the influence of powerfully emerging globalization tendencies. What is being evolved seems to be a need-based social movement with a rich political content.

References

1 Stjernsward, J. (2005). Community participation in palliative care. *Indian Journal of Palliative Care* **11**, 111–117.

2 Gupta, H. (2004). How basic is palliative care? *International Journal of Palliative Nursing* **10**, 600–601.

3 Graham, F. and Clark, D. (2005). Addressing the basics of palliative care. *International Journal of Palliative Nursing* **11**, 36–39.

4 Stjernsward, J. (2007). Palliative Care: The Public Health Strategy. *Journal of Public Health Policy* **28**, 42–55.

5 Clemens, *et al.* (2007). Palliative Care in Developing Countries: What are the important issues? *Palliative Medicine* **21**, 173–175.

6 Raj, K.N., *et al.* (1975). Poverty, unemployment and development policy - a case study of selected issues with reference to Kerala. New York, UN.

7 Ekbal, B. (2000). People's campaign for decentralized planning and the health sector in Kerala, Issue paper, People's Health Assembly. http://phmovement.org/pdf/pubs/phmpubsekbal.pdf

8 Varatharajan, D. (2004). Provision of health care by the government. *Indian Journal of Medical Ethics* **2**(No. 4).

9 George, Asish T. (2005). 'Good health at low cost: How good and how low?' *Economic & Political Weekly* June 18.

10 Levesque, JeanFrédéric, Slim, Haddad, Narayana, Delampady and Fournier, Pierre. (2006). Outpatient care utilization in urban Kerala, India. *Health Policy and Planning* **21**(No.4), 289–301.

11 Rajagopal, M.R. and Kumar, S. (1999). A model for delivery of palliative care in India – the Calicut experiment. *Journal of Palliative Care* **15**, 44–49.

12 Burn, G.L. (1996). Progress of palliative care in India. *Progressive Palliative Care* **4**, 161–162.

13 Rajagopal, M.R. and Palat, G. (2002). Kerala, India: status of cancer pain relief and palliative care. *Journal of Pain and Symptom Management* **24**, 191–193.

14 Ajithakumari, K., Kumar, S. and Rajagopal, M.R. (1997). Palliative home care – the Calicut experience. *Palliative Medicine* **11**, 451–454.

15 Kumar, S. (2007). Kerala, India: a regional community-based palliative care model. *Journal of Pain and Symptom Management* **33**, 623–627.

16 Declaration of Alma-Ata. International conference on primary health care, Alma-Ata, USSR, 6–12 September 1978. Available from http://www.euro.who.int/AboutWHO/Policy/200108271. Accessed April 23, 2008.

17 Morgan, L.M. (2001). Community participation in health: perpetual allure, persistent challenge. *Health Policy Plan* **16**(3), 221–230.

18 Nelson, N., Wright, S. (1995). Power and participatory development: theory and practice. London, I.T. Publications.

19 Sallnow, L. and Chenganakkattil, S. (2005). The role of religious, social and political groups in palliative care in northern Kerala. *Indian Journal of Palliative Care* **11**, 10–14.

20 Kumar, S. (2006). Poverty shouldn't mean poor quality palliative care. *Insights in Health* **8**, 6.

21 Desai, M. (2005). Indirect British rule, state formation, and welfarism in Kerala, India, 1860-1957 *Social Science History* **29**(3), 457–488.

22 Government of Kerala GO(P). 109/2008/ H& FWD Dated 15.4.2008.

Glossary of terms

Chief Executive/Chief Executive Officer: this is the recognized term for the most senior member of staff, responsible and reporting to the Board of Directors/ Governors/Trustees whose task is to oversee the implementation of the decisions and policies of that body.

Community palliative care service: several reasons lie behind the decision to change the traditional term 'home care service' to 'community palliative care service'. It recognizes that people under care in the community may be in their own homes or those of relatives or in nursing homes. Now that there are so many agencies helping the ill or disabled people at home it acknowledges that this care is palliative. Finally, it differentiates this service from those offering domestic help.

Community palliative care services caring for people at home are sometimes termed 'domiciliary services'.

Day Hospice: the term describes a facility for patients under care in the community, who are brought for a few hours each week to a centre, often attached to a hospice/ palliative care unit. There they receive clinical care and usually have the opportunity to see a specialist nurse, doctor or social worker, receive physiotherapy, occupational and art therapy, and enjoy the support of others in a similar situation to themselves.

It should not be confused with 'Day centre', a term more usually reserved for facilities run by the Social Services in the United Kingdom for the elderly, frail, and handicapped.

Day care: this term describes care given to patients attending a hospital/hospice/ palliative care unit on a day basis rather than having to be admitted for such care. For example, there is day-care surgery, day-care oncology, day-care investigations, day-care cardiac catheterization, amongst others.

Doctors: a recently qualified doctor in the United Kingdom is known as a Junior House Officer; in North America, a Resident. A fully trained specialist in the United Kingdom is known as a physician; in North America, an Internist. In the United Kingdom we refer to General Practitioners (GPs); in North America these doctors are known as Family Doctors or Family Physicians (FPs). Worldwide, there is a development towards the term Primary Care Doctor to include GPs, FPs, and all doctors who are the first contact for patients.

Complementary therapies: these are treatments which, while not part of traditional, mainstream medicine, nevertheless complement that care. Examples of complementary therapies sometimes offered in palliative care services include hypnotherapy, aromatherapy, reflexology, reiki, homeopathy, and therapeutic massage.

Homemaker: the person whose prime responsibility is to care for the home and the children. The term must not be confused with what in the United Kingdom is known as a 'Home Help'—someone employed by a statutory or private agency to shop, cook, and do domestic work for those unable to do so for themselves.

Hospice: as explained in Chapter 1, a 'hospice' and a 'palliative care service' are the same thing. 'Hospice' is the word better known by the general public whilst 'palliative care' is the term adopted by health-care professionals because it describes the work done in such a service. In the United States of America 'hospice' is more usually used to describe the philosophy of care rather than the building or service where it is provided.

Matron: it is synonymous with chief nurse, nursing director, head of nursing, director of nursing.

Medical centre: in the United Kingdom, a medical centre is usually the 'surgery' where primary healthcare is provided by general practitioners, community nurses, and professionals allied to medicine. In this book, it is the term applied in Australia to a hospital.

Non-malignant diseases: this term embraces the many diseases that are eventually fatal and which need palliative care but which are not related to cancer. Examples of non-malignant diseases encountered in palliative care units are end-stage cardiac and respiratory diseases, renal disease, AIDS, and many of the rare incurable conditions afflicting children.

Nurse Grades: Nursing Auxiliary is the same as a Nurse Aid in United States of America; Staff Nurse is the same as a Registered Nurse in United States of America. Sister: this is the term for the most senior nurse running a ward in a hospital or in a Health Centre.

Palliative medicine: there are many definitions of palliative 'care' (the term used when describing the care given by nurses or the palliation team as a whole) and palliative 'medicine' (the term used when describing the care given by doctors). The most succinct definition is: *Palliative medicine is the care of people with active, progressive, and far-advanced illness and a short life expectancy, for whom the focus of care is the quality of life.*

Pastoral care worker: this somewhat cumbersome term describes anyone, ordained or not ordained, who caters to the spiritual and religious needs of patients and families. It was coined to avoid terms associated with specific religions or denominations. Titles used range from chaplain and padre to pastoral assistant.

Professions allied to medicine (PAMs): included in this term are occupational therapy, physiotherapy, music therapy, art therapy, drama therapy, stoma therapy, dietetics and nutrition, clinical pharmacy, clinical psychology, and complementary therapy.

Physiotherapists: sometimes known out with the United Kingdom as kinesiotherapists or physical therapists.

Specialist palliative care: this is palliative care provided by a professional—doctor, nurse, pharmacist, pastoral care worker—who is accredited as a specialist by their professional body, having undertaken requisite advanced professional training in palliative care. By early 2002, it was a recognized specialty in the United Kingdom, Australia, New Zealand, Hong Kong, Sweden, and Romania.

Tertiary referral teaching hospital: hospitals where undergraduate and postgraduate doctors and nurses are trained are termed 'teaching hospitals'. Most have highly specialized facilities for patients who have been referred by their primary care doctors (GPs) to hospitals and then been referred on again to these specialist centres, hence the term 'tertiary referral'.

Voluntary Service Manager (VSM): this is the preferred title used in this book for the person more traditionally called the Volunteer Co-ordinator or Co-ordinator of Volunteers.

Index